What Dr. Cosby achieves in this book is nothing short of incredible. His writing style and stories (that is, Cosby's Corner) are witty and captivating, retaining our attention.

—MIKE PHILLIPS
FITNESS TRAINER TO THE STARS

Dr. Cosby's writing is thought provoking, inspiring, educational, motivational, and captivating. This is a book that we believe should be in every family library, read cover to cover, and applied daily to become complete and find your ultimate health.

—GAIL DEVERS
WORLD RECORD HOLDER AND MULTI-GOLD OLYMPIC
AND WORLD CHAMPION WINNER

Dr. Braxton Cosby has been an integral part of developing the fitness strategy of the Put Up Your Dukes Foundation with his key roles in the development of Chachersize for Men and as a cohost of *Ask the Fat Doctors*.

—JAMIE D. DUKES
COHOST OF *ASK THE FAT DOCTORS*,
AUTHOR, NFL NETWORK AND RADIO PERSONALITY

FAT FREE
for Life

FAT FREE for Life

BRAXTON COSBY, DPT

SILOAM

Most CHARISMA HOUSE BOOK GROUP products are available at special quantity discounts for bulk purchase for sales promotions, premiums, fund-raising, and educational needs. For details, write Charisma House Book Group, 600 Rinehart Road, Lake Mary, Florida 32746, or telephone (407) 333-0600.

FAT FREE FOR LIFE by Braxton Cosby, DPT
Published by Siloam
Charisma Media/Charisma House Book Group
600 Rinehart Road
Lake Mary, Florida 32746
www.charismahouse.com

Unless otherwise noted, all Scripture quotations are taken from the Modern English Version. Copyright © 2014 by Military Bible Association. Used by permission. All rights reserved.

Cover design by Lisa Rae McClure
Design Director: Justin Evans

Visit the author's website at www.braxtoncosby.com.

Library of Congress Cataloging-in-Publication Data:
Cosby, Braxton.
  Fat free for life / by Braxton Cosby. -- First edition.
      pages cm
  ISBN 978-1-62136-992-9 (trade paper) -- ISBN 978-1-62136-993-6 (e-book)
  1. Weight loss--Religious aspects--Christianity. 2. Obesity--Religious aspects--Christianity. 3. Health--Religious aspects--Christianity. I. Title.
  RM222.2.C6452 2015
  613.2'5--dc23
                              2014036748

First edition

16 17 18 19 20 — 9 8 7 6 5 4 3 2 1
Printed in the United States of America

This book is dedicated to all of the people out there who are fighting to save lives every day by bringing more awareness to the epidemic of obesity and the disease of excess weight. Those educators, instructors, trainers, nutritionists, therapists, clinicians, and physicians who understand the devastating effects of obesity and the comorbidities that accompany it; you are to be honored for what you do.

I also dedicate this book to the readers who have taken the challenge and decided to allow me to help you in this journey back to ultimate health. Within these pages is the experience, dedication, research, and prayerful instruction of a man that truly wants to see each and every one of you take hold of your lives and be the best you possible.

To my family: Shontel you are so special and important to me; my three princesses, Selene, Sienna, and Sophia, you are the gems in the crown that I wear daily; to my mother, Sharon, who is and will always be an ever present cheerleader and inspiration for me; and to the entire Cosby clan—my big brother, Bryce, father, Robert, Uncle Russell and Aunt Clem, Kenneth, Kelvin, Kandra, Evin, Erika, Ensa, Erin, Aunt Camille and the one and only, Uncle Bill Cosby. The opportunities you have handed me and every person striving to reach their goals are monumental.

And thank you to my Charisma House family for accompanying me on this journey to deliver a book to the masses that I am hopeful will teach and inspire everyone, everywhere to take control of their health. Special thanks to my editor, Jevon: you have been a godsend. Thank you for helping shape this manuscript into the book it is today.

ACKNOWLEDGMENTS

I WOULD LIKE TO take this moment to acknowledge all the many accomplishments I've earned over the rewarding years of my life, and fully and humbly give all the glory and praise to the King of kings who resides in heaven and keeps a watchful eye over me and those I love. I could never do anything without the hand of God and His mighty Son, Jesus Christ.

CONTENTS

FOREWORD

THIS BOOK WILL transform the way you think about three main areas of your life: spirit, mind, and body. Dr. Braxton Cosby has amazing insight into why people struggle with being able to successfully conquer unhealthy eating habits. Most people lose a little weight, but unfortunately later gain it back. Others try to adopt a positive mental attitude to shift their thinking in a different direction. The problem is not weight gain or loss or whether you try to be positive; it's developing a workable, consistent, easy-flowing lifestyle that sustains you and keeps you functioning at your highest level with the added benefit of a long, healthy life. It takes learning how to develop yourself in all three areas—spirit, mind, and body.

Through reading this book, your spiritual life will change. You will find yourself at a higher level of intimate communion with God. Then, how you think will start to permanently transform in critical areas. While this transformation is taking place, you will find yourself desiring to make better decisions in life, including what and how you eat. In these areas you need wisdom that comes from a trained, balanced approach to how and what we eat.

Dr. Braxton Cosby is the best I have ever seen in pulling all three of these areas—spirit, mind, and body—together. The contents of this book will alter your course, change your thinking, and ultimately change your destiny for the good. I speak often of being a work in progress, saying, "What I have is good, it's just incomplete." You don't have to be a disaster case to need this book. What *you* have is good, it's just incomplete! This book will take you to a different level of understanding and move you on a clear path to supernatural breakthrough. Dr. Cosby's insight will open your mind to things that will be unleashed for the sake of destiny.

—BISHOP FRITZ MUSSER
SENIOR PASTOR, TABERNACLE INTERNATIONAL CHURCH
LAWRENCEVILLE, GEORGIA

Introduction

BREAKING CYCLES
OF DEFEAT

THERE IS A serious problem currently trending in the United States. Beyond the failings of the economy, housing, and employment situations, there is a more insidious undertow that is threatening to destroy humanity. It's the prevalence of excess weight or obesity. The epidemic is spreading fast, and the secondary effect of carrying excess weight is seriously hindering our ability to effectively help ourselves and others. Here are some compelling statistics released by the Centers for Disease Control and Prevention:

1. More than two-thirds of adults are either overweight or obese (BMI greater than 25).[1]

2. More than one-third are truly considered obese (BMI greater than 30).[2]

3. Less than one-third are considered to be at a healthy weight (BMI between 18.5–24.9).[3]

As a matter of fact, anyone carrying a BMI (body mass index) greater than thirty is significantly at risk of suffering a heart attack, stroke, or developing diabetes, among other diseases.

That's alarming. To put it into a better perspective, look around the room you are sitting in right now. Find a person to your left and right. One of the three of you is overweight and one of you is obese. If the other two are neither...guess who may be either/or?

But what do these numbers mean to the average person? There are a few assumptions I'd like to point out. For one, people are becoming more sedentary in their lifestyles. The boom in the electronics market (making life very convenient to stay home), the increase in global warming (who wants to go outside anyway?), and the popularity of the fast-food industry have all contributed in one way or another to the steady rise in Americans becoming overweight.

Another reason is people are not controlling the amount of food they are consuming. Going back for seconds, overeating and drinking, and the lack of monitoring the amount of additives will increase caloric intake.

> Fifty percent of all adults who begin an exercise program discontinue within the first six months.

Last is the assumption that there's nothing more you can do. You've tried to stop eating, you've done all the crazy diets, you've wired your mouth shut, you've joined the gym, and you've even wrapped a chain around your refrigerator, but none of it has worked. You've somehow still been able to find a way to pack on the pounds. As a matter of fact, after these attempts you actually gained more weight than you had before you even started.

You're not alone. Many people have experienced this phenomenon. I call it *the cycles of defeat*. Fear not, help is here!

Did you know that 50 percent of all adults who begin an exercise program discontinue within the first six months?[4] As alarming as this statistic is, in my mind, it begs to ask the question: Is society losing the fight against obesity just because we are growing more and more lazy or are there other factors involved in our insidious passage into sickness?

Relatively speaking, it appears that inactivity is a major contributing factor. While on the other hand, regular physical activity is nationally and internationally recognized for its role in preventing several chronic conditions, including heart disease, hypertension, type II diabetes, osteoporosis, and certain site-specific cancers.[5]

So, what's the solution? you may ask. Is it just about encouraging people to get off their butts and move more? If it were that simple, we wouldn't be in this predicament, and furthermore, you wouldn't be here reading this introduction. Right? So there has to be something else. What other aspect of motivation is missing? I mean, a lot of you have done it for your family, yourself, and because your doctor recommended it. But you still came up empty, back on the other side of the scale. You know, the one that says, "Oh, no you didn't!" when you step off the scale. I want to add one last motivational component to managing your weight that I'm sure you may not have tried yet. How about a godly one?

What God Called You to Do

You may have asked the question: "What does God have for me?" or "What is His plan for my life?" For most people, it starts with acceptance—acceptance of the truth that God has a specific plan to use you to do great things. This plan for your life is one that incorporates not only a mission to receive blessings for yourself (through building a closer relationship with God in all aspects of your life), but also a directive to bring others into intimacy with God, through His Son, Jesus Christ. Any one believer can say that he knows of Him. That's easy. We read His Word, we attend church, we even pray to Him, but can we truly say we really know Him? It starts with a relationship.

Somebody once asked me how I define the word relationship. Honestly, I was not sure. I felt that in order to build a relationship with someone you must have a commitment to believe in or trust a person, to understand that a person has your best interests in mind. But I really didn't have a definite answer to the question. The person shared with me that to have a relationship means to know someone's voice.

To hear God's voice in your life on a daily basis means you have a relationship with Him. This can be confusing to most, because everyone hears voices in their heads, but how do you know that it's God speaking to you?

> God has a specific plan to use you to do great things.

To know someone is not to hear that person's voice and to understand what you hear, but to be able to discern that voice from any other voice in the world. If a good friend called you on the phone one day and said hello, immediately you would know who that person was without hearing his name. That's because you have established a relationship over time and you are very familiar with him. You recognize the pitch, tone, and volume at which he speaks. When he is happy, sad, upset, or excited, you can tell. The variable inflection in his voice is indicative of the mood he is in, even before you ask him.

The same should be true with God. When He calls you, are you able to hear His voice? You would if you've spoken to Him on a regular basis, because you have endeavored to truly invest in that relationship to know the Father.

I struggled with that myself. I realized that the voices in my head were in competition with one another for my attention. They told me to do certain things, they suggested that I follow a certain path, and they even spoke to me when I was about to make the right or wrong decisions. But how was I to know which one was God speaking to me?

The truth is, I was playing a game with God. I used Him like a tool. I pulled Him out of the tool chest when I needed Him and put Him back when I felt that I could do things on my own. It was a partnership based on needs and wants.

When that type of relationship began to fail me (and it did countless times), I had to take another route. I began to press into God more. Read His Word, search its truths, and ask Him to speak to me on a daily, regular, uninterrupted basis. And I can admittedly say I began to recognize His voice.

I began to understand His will and purpose for my life, and I was convinced, persuaded, and unequivocally led to believe that God had set me aside for a purpose. This was because I started to build a foundation on the faith that I was no different from the heroes in the Bible. God's Word tells of when God called simple people to do amazing feats (part the Red Sea, shut the mouths of lions, hold back the rain, and bring the dead back to life). I realized that I was from the same lineage as those people. They are my spiritual family, and all I had to do was honor God, hold Him to His promises, and simply believe.

What He Called Me to Do

If you're reading this and you are interested in trying to build your relationship with God so that you can tap into the power necessary to overcome the cycles of defeat, you must first answer these questions:

1. Do you know His voice?

2. Are you sure that God has a special calling on your life?

3. Are you willing to answer the calling?

If you're not sure, then you too might not be in relationship with Him. You, like me, may know *of* Him but not know Him. And out of everything I have come to understand, I'm convinced that the one thing God wants us to do is have a relationship with Him, one that goes beyond religion and delves into a spiritual connection with the Holy Trinity—the Father, the Son, and the Holy Spirit. The only way to get there is a daily walk with Him.

I was called by God to write this book, and I was both thrilled and humbled by the opportunity to do so. I wanted to use my experience and knowledge to galvanize people to take control of their health. Stop losing the battles and being discouraged, and start waging war against the enemy. He has entrusted me with the vision.

We are spirit beings who have a soul and live in a body. Therefore, in order to live in the fullness of all God has for us, we must strengthen each of these components of our being.

Our spirit pants for God like the deer pants for water. It is in constant communion with God, searching the deep thoughts of God and providing divine insight and instruction for us.

The soul is the emotive part of our being. It is the *brain center*. Our actions, reactions, and responses originate here. The gateway to the soul is through the eyes. What goes in through the eyes, passes directly into the soul. It's the visual connection of the outside world, the mind, and the soul. They are connected, interlinked in such a way that information instantly downloads into all three, and we either believe the information as the truth or we disseminate it as fiction.

Therefore, it is important for us to evaluate what we *feed* ourselves on various platforms: television, reading, computers, and our plates. You love chocolate cake, can't resist taking another forkful even though you know your stomach is sending the message of satiety—turn away. Your soul will thank you for it. If you are trying to eat right, don't go down the aisle of the grocery store where the cakes, cookies, and other sugar-filled snacks are. You've already established the connection between your stomach and your soul for foods like these. It's time to reprogram your soul's desires and replace them with what your body needs.

> Stop losing the battles and being discouraged, and start waging war against the enemy.

Then there is the physical, your body. It is that object in the mirror that you are either fully satisfied with, or have some reservations of showing off at the beach in that two-piece bikini (ladies) or Speedo (men). Well, maybe that was a stretch, but I'm sure you get the picture. I challenge you to consider that lump of flesh in a new mind-set—as a lump of clay, able to be molded and reconfigured in the fullness of what God intended.

Many of us lose the battle of the bulge because we fail to address all three of these. We work out like crazy (the physical) but we neglect the mental and spiritual, which inevitably leads us back down the path to loss. Our minds are weak, our spiritual relationship is broken, and we blindly cling to the notion that looking in the mirror and focusing only on the physical will make long-lasting, positive change. The wounds of soul and spirit are still open and vulnerable, allowing the enemy to take hold of us and send waves of discouragement and doubt.

> It's time to reprogram your soul's desires and replace them with what your body needs.

I have been instructed to help. God called me to write this book so that people can once again use the power of God like the prophets of old did. They accomplished great feats through faith, *and you can too*! This book will provide insight into utilizing God's power through testimony (mental), inspirational word (spiritual), and statistical evidence-based facts (physical) to educate, encourage, and inspire people to not only understand His will for their lives, but to break the cycles of defeat that are holding you back from achieving all that God has to offer.

What Can We Do Together?

This three-headed approach to reversing the cycles of defeat will give you the tools to empower you to overcome the things that are holding you back. More specifically, this book will help to motivate you to be a healthier you so that God may be able to use you to do His will. Those God called were ready and willing, and physically, mentally, and spiritually able to do so because they were healthy.

As you read the pages of this book, ask God to open your mind, heart, and spirit so that you are able to receive what He has given me to pass on to you. Decide that you will no longer be a victim of yourself. Be convinced that up to this point you have been holding you back, and it's time to remove the old self and walk in the new self that God has *been* and *is* calling you to be. With the infusion of the new man, you will be able to walk in victory, be healthy, and allow your testimony to inspire and encourage others to do great things.

Interspersed throughout the chapters of this book you will find special sections I have called "Cosby's Corner." These sections are filled with my personal challenges to you as you walk through this journey to break the cycles of defeat that have held you back from victorious living.

In Luke 1:28–38, Mary (the mother of Jesus) said it best when the angel of God came to her concerning the birth of Jesus. Mary didn't question what the angel said. She responded by saying, "I am the servant of the Lord. May it be unto me according to your word" (v. 38). I plead with you today; let it be unto you, according to the rich, everlasting Word of God.

> It's time to remove the old self and walk in the new self that God has been and is calling you to be.

Chapter 1

CLAIM SUCCESS FOR A NEW SEASON

T HIS CHAPTER WILL begin to reveal the steps to move from victim to victor as you learn to move to a new season that brings success in the three important areas of soul (mind), spirit, and body. We will look at each of these areas, focusing on the path to victory in each. In each of these areas, you must begin by learning to recognize the voice of God as He speaks to you and empowers you for the journey.

Use Your Mind to Shape a New Identity

As you begin to understand the importance of training your mind to partner with the voice of God as He leads you into a new, victorious identity, I want to start with a personal testimony. Imagine that you are with me in this experience that led me to a new victorious mental attitude.

I'm in the gym, going through my regular workout routine, performing an incline chest press, and all of a sudden I feel a

---

sharp pain to my left collarbone. I put down the dumbbells in my hands and slowly rotate my left shoulder forward and back. The pain seems to subside for a moment, so I continue on with my workout.

Later on I try another exercise, this time dumbbell over-head press. The throbbing, lingering pain continues to per-sist as I continue to add weights. With each repetition I feel it driving into me, stabbing at me like a sharp knife. I shrug it off and attribute it to old age (an over-the-hill athlete at the age of thirty-six), ignore it, and proceed to complete the rest of my workout, utilizing a spotter to help me through when necessary.

I go home at night and treat myself conservatively with ice and stretching. After falling asleep, I awaken to find that the pain is still there. It hides underneath my collarbone and cuts at me like a knife. Every time I lift my arm over my head to put on my shirt, the pain increases. This annoys me to no end, but not enough to prevent me from continuing my workout.

So I go back to the gym the next day and work out again, this time focusing on my biceps and triceps. Thankfully, no pain this time, so I take my rest day and return the following day for chest, back, and shoulders. And guess who's waiting for me? The insidious pain under my collarbone!

This time when I reach home, it's pill-popping time—Advil and Tylenol, along with an application of ice again. Then I stretch like crazy, praying for the day that things will return back to normal.

Time goes on, actually over a period of six weeks now. But that nagging pain that only came on when I lifted my hands over my head has advanced into something new: a cracking, drilling, burning ache that exists when I do anything other than lie down. I feel it when I sit at my desk to write notes during patient care. It accompanies me in my car rides to and from work. Simple tasks such as reaching for a box of cereal from a high shelf or cleaning my bathroom mirror exacerbate the painful symptoms.

I'm now growing frustrated, but I have yet to determine that I need to see a physician for a second opinion. It's manageable, right? At least that's what I think.

Frustrated more than ever now, I decide to seek spiritual help. I pray to God, pressing into Him and asking Him to show me what I need to do in order to overcome my pain and move forward with my life. I'm a physical therapist. This is an embarrassment. Heat, ice, electrical stimulation, and ultrasound have not made a dent in my pain.

Then it finally happened to me. God spoke. He told me that it wasn't my pain anymore that was controlling me—it was my fear of the pain. He was right, as always. I hesitated when I needed to lift my arm. I cringed at the idea of lying on my left side. And I reluctantly used my left arm when helping my wife take the groceries out of the car. My fear had now become my stronghold, and I needed help. I had addressed the physical, and when my methods failed, my soul became disheartened. I needed a spiritual intervention.

But that's where God came in. I was determined that He could heal me, but it would take an intervention at all three aspects—spirit, soul, and body—working together synchronously to effectively bring about my total healing.

I started in the spiritual, asking God to bring healing into my life—specifically to that small muscle underneath my clavicle (subclavius muscle). It was responsible for the subtle rotation that needed to occur to allow my arm to rise over my head past ninety degrees.

After my prayer, I was convinced that my healing had started. I began to address the physical component, performing exercises specifically targeted at healing that muscle. As a pain crept back in with each repetition, I knew my next step would entail controlling my emotion of fear. That's where my soul came in.

> God reassured me that everything I needed to succeed was already within me.

I performed each exercise in the mirror, watching myself carefully, checking my form and technique. With a light grimace plastered across my face, I fought through the pain, performing each shoulder flexion and diagonal adduction exercise under control, providing my soul the positive feedback it needed to establish that I *could* execute the movement in the presence of fear. I could overcome my pain because I believed that God could heal me. As I continued to have faith, God reassured me that everything I needed to succeed was already within me. It only took the belief that I was in control of my emotional responses with the assurance that God had started the healing process.

Within one week, the thing that had tortured me and enslaved my mind had been removed. The pain, along with the fear, was wiped away and was replaced with victory. I now reestablished God as a healer. My new season of overcoming pain was now here.

How do you get here with me? It's easy. Shape your identity. Before you walk into your new season, you need to establish who you really are. For starters, let me tell you something: YOU ARE NOT FAT! On a personal level, I've never been called fat before in my entire life. I've always been on the slim side. But I can relate to having an identity crisis when it comes to my weight. Being told that I was skinny enough to Hula Hoop in a Cheerio was tragic enough. But I always wondered how it felt to be called fat. I could only imagine how overweight individuals feel when someone calls them that, or when they see someone else who everyone considers to be skinny. Do they feel downcast, ashamed, and riddled with self-pity that only makes them cycle into more of a downward spiral, emotionally eating more and more in order to satisfy some inner craving to be accepted? I would, wouldn't you?

Why do people overeat? Some people are so emotionally frightened that they crave food as an escape. Others overeat because of cultural norms. Some people are victims of their own family values that have taught them to always clean their plates, and to consume foods that are

> Before you walk into your new season, you need to establish who you really are.

high in saturated fats because that is all they can afford. Socioeconomics plays a key factor in the quality of the food people eat. We now know that it's not just the quantity of the food we eat that dictates our weight gain, but the quality of the food. In some cases, quality is more of a factor.

I know I can't change the world overnight concerning these two circumstances, but I want to implore you to join hands with me and make an attempt to stop viewing overweight people as fat. People are not fat. They may have an excess amount of fatty tissue, but they are not fat. Overweight folks have muscles, bones, and, most of all, feelings, just like those who are not overweight. It may seem like a matter of semantics, but people have to begin thinking differently if they are to overcome their shortcomings.

If you are a part of an overweight family, you are not fat. You have fat on you, yes, but you are an angel, sent from God, with a God-given purpose. You have the ability within you to accomplish so much more than you have done so far. It starts with getting your health right, then with moving on to being used to help others. If you are able to accomplish those things, then the sky is the limit. Don't be a victim of the identity that society has placed on you. Your identity is so much more than a visual image or a set of digits on a scale.

> Your identity is so much more than a visual image or a set of digits on a scale.

COSBY'S CORNER
Hang 'em High

It's a good idea to hang your fitness goals somewhere that you can see them. Don't put them on your office desk or inside your clothing drawer where they become fodder for the trash can when you get the inclination to do some spring cleaning.

No. Make them a tangible visual by placing them in a place where you can see them daily—maybe taped on your bathroom mirror or hung on your closet door. You have to make them real, not just a floating idea that pops into your head once or twice during the day.

Your goals have to become a reality to you. You should see them in the morning when you wake up and before you go to bed. Actualization of a dream is the first step to seeing it come true.

Put them in a place that detours you from continuing bad behavior. Um, maybe . . . I don't know . . . some place random like . . . the refrigerator. Yeah! Plant your flag dead center in the enemy's battlefield. That is usually in your mind, right? But when it comes to fighting the war against eating, the true war is fought right at the space between you and the food.

Why not make multiple copies and place them all around the house? The kitchen cabinet, snack drawer (don't tell me you don't have one—candy, candy, candy), and even the place where you put your keys once you make it home. It will be a good reminder of what you are working toward before you make that late night food run because times are getting hard.

Another reason to place fitness goals out in the open is because it encourages people to be all up in your business. That's right! You need someone to know what you are up to. The more people who know about the journey you are embarking on, the better it will be for you in the end.

Trust me here. You know why? Because people are nosy. They like nothing more than having something to talk about . . . and it probably will be you more often than not. They'll say things like: "I can't believe what he's doing, going on a diet. You know that man doesn't have an ounce of self-control. When they handed that out in heaven, he was standing in line next to the snow-cone machine." Or, "Yeah, girl, she's trying to work out now. Um, hmm. The only running she ever does is run her mouth."

But relax, relax. This is going to work in your favor. You know how they say it takes a village to raise a child? Well, it takes a nation to stop someone from scarfing down bowls of chocolate ice cream—scratch that—a hot fudge brownie with chocolate ice cream on top of it, covered with nuts and layering whipped cream all over it.

Now I'm talking, right?

Take a minute to wipe the drool off my book and get your head back in the game. Accountability is the key ingredient here. The more folks know what's going on, the more they can motivate you to stay the course (even if the motivation is coming from a place of negativity). You need everything imaginable to help you out at this point. I'm just saying . . .

■■■

Empower Your Spirit for the Journey

How can you begin to walk in a new season for your life? You can empower your spirit through the Word of God. Let's take a look at a few scriptures from the Word where God is calling a new season for His followers.

Psalm 1:3 reads:

> He will be like a tree planted by the rivers of water, that brings forth its fruit in its season; its leaf will not wither, and whatever he does will prosper.

God has a reason for using this analogy of the tree. King Solomon said that there's a time to every purpose under heaven. It is important to understand that life is cyclical, and that everyone has their moments on top and on the bottom. But the difference between being the *victor* and being the *victim* is that the victors push that timetable closer together. With each loss they lift themselves up from the ground and battle back to being winners. They do not pout, hang their heads low, and wade in the murky waters of subjugation.

They make their way to dry land, plant their feet on solid ground, establish a firm foundation, and march their way back up—seeking victory, seeking a new season in their lives that embodies the concept of being a tree planted by streams of water, a tree that will bend in the breeze of tribulation, but that will not break. Its roots are deep, taking

> Everyone has their moments on top and on the bottom. But the difference between being the victor and being the victim is that the victors push that timetable closer together.

in the daily nourishment from the life-giving waters of God. And if that tree stands firm to the promise of another daily provision, it will yield fruit in the season that God has already predestined.

In Mark chapter 10 verses 46–52 Jesus met the blind man where he was, because he knew that the season for change was at hand. Let's look at what happened.

> Then they came to Jericho. And as He went out of Jericho with His disciples and a great number of people, blind Bartimaeus, the son of Timaeus, sat along the way begging. When he heard that it was Jesus of Nazareth, he began to cry out, "Jesus, Son of David, have mercy on me!" Many ordered him to keep silent. But he cried out even more, "Son of David, have mercy on me!"

Jesus stood still and commanded him to be called. So they called the blind man, saying, "Be of good comfort. Rise, He is calling you." Throwing aside his garment, he rose and came to Jesus. Jesus answered him, "What do you want Me to do for you?" The blind man said to Him, "Rabbi, that I might receive my sight." Jesus said to him, "Go your way. Your faith has made you well." Immediately he received his sight and followed Jesus on the way.

What's profound in this passage of Scripture is the faith that Bartimaeus had. He didn't waver between doubt and failure. He was convinced that Jesus could do whatever He said He could. He knew that he wanted to receive his sight more than anything else. His determination to see was far greater than his fear of failure. When Jesus asked him, "What do you want Me to do for you?" Bartimaeus told Him, specifically, what he wanted. Jesus established that it was not anything external that healed him; it was the faith that dwelled within him that healed him. It was an instantaneous occurrence.

> Ask God for the strength to do what you need to in order to bring about a mental, spiritual, and physical healing. The season is now!

We have to live within that same principle of healing. *Now* is the time for victory. Now is the time to take back what has been stolen from you. You have let the enemy blind you for far too long. If you have the faith to ask God to take you into a season of victory, then you will immediately be on your way. This is your season to take control of your health. Stop sitting by the side of the road wallowing in self-pity, suffering from a loser's mentality. Don't let God pass you by anymore. You can stand to your feet, approach the Son of God, and let Him know what you want. Proclaim it boldly. Ask Him for the strength to do what you need to in order to bring about a mental, spiritual, and physical healing. The season is now!

Provide Your Body With the Tools of Success

Researchers continue to explore the effects of positive thinking and optimism on health. Health benefits that positive thinking may provide include:

> Positive thinking may ensure success even more than eliminating something you have been eating.

- Increased life span

- Lower rates of depression

- Lower levels of distress

- Greater resistance to the common cold

- Better psychological and physical well-being

- Reduced risk of death from cardiovascular disease

- Better coping skills during hardships and times of stress

This supports the important effects of having a positive outlook on life. One of the most important tools you can give your body is the optimistic attitude of your mind. Positive thinking may ensure success even more than eliminating something you have been eating. Many studies have shown that overweight individuals who believe they can be successful lose more pounds than less positive dieters. You must believe that no matter what, *you will succeed.*

Arlene K. Unger, clinical psychologist and wellness coach, suggests the following important tips for partnering your mind with your body for successful and sustained weight loss.

1. **Begin with baby steps**—Start with substituting one food item at a time. Remember self-confidence begets success, and success begets self-mastery, begets self-confidence.

2. **Focus on behavior change, not weight loss**—You will reach your goals by changing behavior, not by losing pounds.

3. **Learn from your mistakes**—Be ready to **try, try again.** Don't look at your relapses as failures, but rather as learning experiences.

4. **Find someone to follow**—Behavior change is more successful when you find an inspired role mode.

5. **Get lots of reinforcement**—There is nothing like getting support from your friends, colleagues, and family.

6. **Concentrate on changing patterns, not your diet regime**—When you feel restricted and deprived it is a natural reaction to rebel.

7. **Reward yourself**—Verbal or actual pats on the back increase your motivation and help you feel strong in facing the next moment.[1]

I've worked as a clinician for more than thirteen years, six of which have been in the geriatric population, and I have seen firsthand the power of a positive outlook to provide the body with the motivation it needs to be successful with the development of new, successful behaviors that ensure success in the area of a healthy body.

There is a direct link between death and frailty in the absence of positive thinking. The relationship between physical and mental health problems begins to blend more over time. The rapid decline of a sick elder is the result of despondency and "giving up."[2] Those individuals who allow themselves to let their circumstances dictate their happiness, lose control, spiraling off into the deadly sequelae of events that ultimately lead to even more sickness. When those individuals focus only on the negative aspects of their lives, it only adds to their struggles, and makes them even more prone to develop an attitude of defeat.

Whether you are young or old, underweight or overweight, active or inactive, if you partner your positive, optimistic spirit with your health-producing behavior modifications you will find the success you are looking for—mind, body, and spirit.

It's like what Paul said:

> Finally, brothers, whatever things are true, whatever things are honest, whatever things are just, whatever things are pure, whatever things are lovely, whatever things are of good report, if there is any virtue, and if there is any praise, think on these things.
> —PHILIPPIANS 4:8

Think on these things! Remember, claiming your season ahead of time sets you up for God to establish you on the path today that will guide you where He intends for you to be. Claiming it (in faith) shows God that you believe and that He is worthy of praise.

Chapter 2

RECOGNIZE AND MOVE PAST YOUR OBSTACLES

O NCE YOU HAVE recognized the importance of making some necessary changes in your life, and have prepared yourself for the journey by understanding the steps we covered in the first chapter, it is now time to identify and move past those things in your mind, body, and spirit that have hindered you from being successful.

Understand Your Mental Barriers

Take the time to identify the things that have been specific hindrances preventing you from accomplishing your health goals. Most people are not sure where to start, but I suggest that you begin right in your own environment or living space. Assess the things that are right before you, distracting and deterring you from putting forth the maximal effort needed to break through. These are your barriers to success. No doubt they will include eating too late at night, consuming large quantities of high calorie foods, and staying away from the gym. These things will seriously destroy any chances of you making a dent in that *spare tire* or of finally emptying out that *junk from inside the trunk.*

Once you identify the things that are stripping you of the power to be successful, then you can remove them and make life changes that facilitate growth in the positive direction. By doing so, you will give yourself leverage to turn the odds in your favor. Your window of success will enlarge, bringing all the target goals you set within your grasp.

I once spoke with a good friend of mine who struggled with weight loss for a long time. She was generally someone that you would see on the street and never think that she would be prone to have weight issues later on in life. In her pre-college years, she weighed in anywhere between one hundred five and one hundred fifteen pounds.

But then things changed. She said it began in college with the *freshman twenty* and progressed from there. Over the years that followed she continued to add more and more weight. It was insidious. She never saw it coming. She'd wake up and look in the mirror, each day maybe adding an ounce here, a pound there, but nothing dramatic enough to make her aware of the gains.

Finally, after ten or so years, there it was. Forty plus pounds of weight gain, staring her right in her face. She became self-conscious and insecure, purposely avoiding pool parties and gatherings that provided opportunities to show *too much.* She had a difficult time dating because of her weight and lack of confidence. Her food had become her comfort, along with her focus on her work.

In her mind, losing weight became a topic of discussion only in circles of close friends in whom she could confide because they may be struggling with the same weight issues themselves. Crash diet after diet, exercise program after exercise program, and even some medical interventions later, she was still there—trapped in the body of a person that she did not recognize.

As she entered her late thirties she decided to make a *real* change. She got hungry for breaking the cycles of defeat in her life. She determined to change her habits and the bad ways that were fostering her losses. She chose to turn them into successes. She began to monitor her caloric intake on a daily basis, establishing a goal of no more than twelve hundred calories per day.

> No crazy diets, no pills, and no shots— just the diligence to follow a routine that was right for you and a will to believe in changing the atmosphere by breaking bad habits for good.

Keeping a daily log was essential. She says that she had to be honest with herself and not merely estimate values but truly account for them. Then she enrolled in a gym, participating in weekly classes to increase her weekly activity to help wake up her metabolism and *ramp* it up. "These two combinations are what really got me going," she says. "I had an *energy* about me that I hadn't felt in a long time."

There was a give and take system in place. On the days that she really needed a high calorie snack fix (like a piece of candy or slice of cake), she knew that she would have to cut out a larger meal for lunch or dinner. There was no time to try and make it up another day. The time to effectually make a change was that day only. "I can remember going to sleep hungry some nights because I had already eaten too many calories," she states, "but as time went by, my body changed, and I adapted to smaller portions."

Now my friend has lost more than fifty pounds in one year's time, and she is feeling and looking great. No crazy diets, no pills, and no shots—just the diligence to follow a routine that was right for her and a will to believe in changing the atmosphere by breaking bad habits for good.

> Rome wasn't built in a day, and neither will your body.

Eating less, moving more, and allowing your body the time it needs to adjust to the new life changes that you are introducing are critical steps in making the drive toward better health. You have to remember this: You added on the weight over a long period of time. Your body has made changes (mostly negative) to adapt to the excess weight. It got used to moving slower, breathing deeper, and shunting blood away from areas that are less active to the ones that are working more, like the stomach, brain, and heart. Thus, it will take time for your body to switch from the sedentary person that you have become to the exercise enthusiast that you want to be. Sore muscles, burning lungs, sweat in parts of your body that have become foreign to you are all par for the course. Let it settle in for a little bit. Rome wasn't built in a day, and neither will your body.

COSBY'S CORNER
Ice Skating Uphill

Ice skating uphill is the quintessential analogy for what most people do when they embark on the course of setting things right concerning their health.

Many people start fitness programs and diets and get all discouraged when the results either don't come fast enough or don't come at all. But everything takes time, folks. It's easy to drift off into the dream world of believing that the weight that took years to put on will somehow just melt away since you finally got serious about doing something. You may be staring impatiently at the free moving hand on the scale as you stand in pulsating expectation. But alas, it just doesn't work like that; nor do you want it to. The truth is that fad diets, fasts, and quick weight loss schemes just don't produce long-lasting results. There's no miracle cure or lightning in a bottle creation that will offset good ole fashioned hard work. And it is hard work, no doubt about it.

I once had an elderly patient who lived in a nursing home who suffered with dementia and a fractured hip. I was treating him for ambulation training after he was fitted with a brand-new hip socket at the hospital. I scheduled to work with him in the morning. After I finished up some paperwork I headed to his room to take him down to the gym. When I got to his room, I was greeted by the most *interesting* smell. (Sidebar: see how interesting is italicized, folks? It means interesting, not just run of the mill interesting. Keep reading.) I gently tapped on his door and entered the room.

Wave after wave of what I can only describe as wet diapers and molded bread blitzed my nostrils, along with a smothering, dank warmth. I found it somewhat hard to breathe, but I became a bit worried when the patient did not respond to my calling his name. I turned the corner of the room to where his bed was positioned and found him bottom naked, standing next to the heater, which was on full blast. He gave me an innocent smile and explained to me that his boxers were soiled, and he had taken the liberty of hand washing and draping them on top of the—wait for it—heater!

I reluctantly turned my head to look at the heater and was greeted by the vision of a light blue, stiff as double-reinforced cardboard, brown-streaked (sorry for the imagery) pair of boxers lying across the vent. I have to admit that I was somewhat relieved, because at least it explained the smell that had curiously haunted my nose for the last few minutes.

What was the reason for this story, other than me selfishly passing on the stalking ghosts of my mental images to you? It's simple. He had a good idea, based on good intentions, but obviously failed to plan appropriately, which resulted in poor execution and, dare I say, stinky results.

Remember people, if you want to do something right, with the most fulfilling experience, and get the most desirable results, you have to properly plan and take the necessary steps that will ensure the most favorable outcomes.

The long road to health is life changing, and once you adopt those healthy practices you are in for some serious victories. No short-cuts, no compromises, and, definitely, no fast tracking. Fast tracking would only cause you to become short-fused in your thinking process, which would make you crave results that were quick and temporal. Such faulty action only sets you up for the all-too-familiar rebounding and yo-yo pounds on, pounds off phenomenon. It lands you in the unflattering position of feeling as if you were caught with your pants down, with all the world watching. Don't be tempted.

Let's face it: Ice skating uphill expends way too much energy and does not guarantee that the reward is worth the effort. I'm just saying...

■■■

Empower Your Spirit With Valuable Biblical Truth

What does the Bible say about the value of having a plan? It actually warns us that it is senseless or improper to do anything without first assessing the situation. In Luke 14:31, Jesus gives it to us in a parable when He says: "Or what king, going to wage war against another king, does not sit down first and take counsel whether he is able with ten thousand to meet him who comes against him with twenty thousand?"

This verse references a king going to do battle against another king. He first considers the possible outcomes based on his odds of success. I imagine he'd ask questions like: "Who am I up against?" "Do I have enough troops?" "Are my men properly trained for battle?" "What is the terrain like where we will be fighting?" "What are my available resources?"

Let me give you a word of advice concerning your new season of health and wellness: You are at war also! You should ask yourself the same questions and answer them accordingly.

1. Who am I up against?

You are up against *yourself!* The biggest resistance you will face is Y-O-U. Brace yourself, the next seventy-two hours after your first day of exercise will be the toughest. You will feel pain in places that you didn't know you even had muscles. Your ability to drag yourself from the bed and get back into the gym will be critical. Your mind and body will cry out for you to stop, but you must press on. Pull the strength from a place deep within and press forward. Trust me, this too will pass.

2. Do I have enough troops?

Yes. You are equipped with everything you need to succeed right now. You are equipped with the power of the Holy Spirit (Acts 1:8). The fact that you are able to get up and face another day is proof that you have arrived in a new season, and everything is coming together for your purpose. Your divine appointment is now.

> We have to recognize that the strength to persevere comes from the heavenly place.

3. Are my men properly trained for battle?

Yes. You have received a spirit of power, strength, and a sound mind (2 Tim. 1:7). You are not a slave to the flesh; you have mastered it through your spiritual inheritance (Gal. 4:7). Jesus conquered the grave and removed all the weapons of the enemy so that you can walk in authority over all principalities (Col. 2:15). That loser's mentality that you once owned is now gone—laid to rest with the other dead things of this world.

4. What is the terrain like where we will be fighting?

You will be fighting on a spiritual battlefield. The Bible tells us in Ephesians 6:12: "For our fight is not against flesh and blood, but against principalities, against powers, against the rulers of the darkness of this world, and against spiritual forces of evil in the heavenly places." Your struggles—at work, in your relationships, your marriage, your relatives, your children, and your time at the gym—are against things unseen by the naked eye. Therefore, we have to recognize that the strength to persevere comes from the heavenly place. We have to call on God to bind those things that war against us so that we can overcome them. That next burning repetition that will get you the results you need is waiting for you, reserved just for you in a spiritual place of healing. But it will not be attained without fighting through those things that are determined to discourage you and keep you subjugated to a defeated mentality.

5. What are my available resources?

Your most valuable resource is the Lord! He will be your strength and shield. Psalm 28:7 captures this by telling us:

> The LORD is my strength and my shield; my heart trusted in Him, and I was helped; therefore my heart rejoices, and with my song I will thank Him.

The Lord will provide both strength and shield for the battle at hand. In this new season you will be able to deliver a blow to the enemy that is so devastating he will have to run and hide. God's shield will protect you from the enemy's return. Even though he will descend upon you and tell you that you are not good enough to finish that set, to jog on that treadmill, and to pass up that delicious piece of cake, you will be protected. And because you are, you will repel the attacks and fight on.

So we have what the Bible says about having a plan, but what about removing these so-called barriers? I like to think of them as shackles. They keep you captive to the old thinking of your mind—the sweet tastes of that sugar, the feeling of that warm bread roll as you take it out of the oven with warm butter melting all over it, and the feeling of that high fructose corn syrup-filled soft drink as it bubbles and fizzes down your throat after a long, stressful day. *Wake up! We are at war here.* Removing these thoughts is just the beginning. We have to replace them with new ones.

The tailor-made path that will lead to your fitness freedom is laid before you, and all you have to do is press in and run.

Remember that the eyes are the pathway to the soul. Your soul has become trained to love those things because that is all it's been bombarded with. Let's switch it up now, change the game a bit. Instead of those scoops of ice-cream, let's try a low calorie frozen yogurt. Still addicted to those cinnamon rolls? Angel food cake might be the answer. Still not convinced? Biblically speaking, Hebrews 12:1–2 may provide some insight:

> Therefore, since we are encompassed with such a great cloud of witnesses, let us also lay aside every weight and the sin that so easily entangles us, and let us run with endurance the race that is set before us. Let us look to Jesus, the author and finisher of our faith, who for the joy that was set before Him endured the cross, despising the shame, and is seated at the right hand of the throne of God.

I love that verse. It describes the landscape for you. You are surrounded by a great cloud of witnesses, heavenly hosts, looking down on you, rooting for you to rise and take hold of the power of God. They are beckoning you to throw off everything—those chains, those doubts, and even some of those friends that will literally get you killed (oh yeah, they eat, you eat...to death) if you don't have the strength to stop. Once you eliminate them, then you are able to run with all perseverance the race that God has marked out for you. The tailor-made path that will lead to your fitness freedom is laid before you, and all you have to do is press in and run. Your spiritual trainer is Jesus. Keep your eyes fixed on Him, and He will continue to perfect your faith. If you need more than just the idea of spiritual witnesses to keep you accountable, recruit friends or join a boot camp. Let someone else hold you to the plan.

This is your fitness plan, your road map to success. It starts with prudent planning and ends with removing obstacles! Don't even think for a moment that a haphazard approach to wellness will enable you to lose a single pound.

Give Your Body *Good* Stressors, Not *Bad* Ones

We've talked briefly about the need to exercise and that exercise is a stress to the body. Most people say they try to avoid stress as much as possible. And for the most part, I agree that things that add unnecessary stress to your life should be avoided. But (and there is always a *but*) exercise is not one of them. I illustrated this in the earlier chapters, emphasizing that exercise is the *good* stress that causes your body to take action, to adapt over time to make the positive changes that you need to meet your fitness potential. This is different from the *bad* stressors.

Things like adverse social conditions, negative life events, relationship hassles, conflicts in the workplace, family illnesses or death, and major life changes are just a few things that really begin to take a toll on the human psyche. You can begin to feel overwhelmed, like you are drowning in a never-ending sea of responsibility. This stress has physical consequences and can be deadly. Elevations in blood pressure occur with the persistent circulation of blood flow to mobilize hormones and fuel working muscles.

Which hormones you ask? Adrenaline and cortisol. They activate the sympathetic part of your autonomic nervous system; the *fight or flight* mechanism that helps to protect you in dangerous times. If you are being run down by a vicious animal, or about to be hit by a car, the sympathetic nervous system secretes these hormones to prepare your body for action.

Adrenaline causes increased spikes in heart rate, respiratory rate, and blood flow. It shifts your body into the next gear, giving you the potential for increased speed and strength. Cortisol, on the other hand, dampens other systems of the body like the immune and digestive systems. It allows more blood to be shunted

> Low-stress individuals have a stronger cardiovascular response to stress, making them less likely to suffer a heart attack or stroke.

to parts of the body that need it like the brain, heart, lungs, and working muscle. This is good for only short periods of time. Continued or chronic stress keeps the amount of these hormones elevated longer than necessary, which brings about negative changes. Imagine, your digestion now begins to be impaired and you have problems going to the bathroom regularly. Then, your immune system is stunted, making you more prone to being sick. This combination alone can be lethal, making you eat less, which will make you lose weight (*stress diet*), but not the right way. Depression sets in soon after, and then you eat the foods that are not good for you (comfort foods) but feel satisfying.

Chronic stress that results from economic hardship and inner-city living has been consistently linked to hypertension (high blood pressure), which could lead to a higher incidence of heart disease. When comparing high-stress individuals

> Substituting one stress (good) for the other (bad) is vital in creating the right atmosphere for success.

to low-stress individuals, low-stress individuals have a stronger cardiovascular response to stress, making them less likely to suffer a heart attack or stroke.[1]

Making the adjustments sooner rather than later is more important than you may think. As time goes by, the body begins to make changes that are somewhat irreversible and your ability to adapt to varying internal or external conditions becomes less flexible—which means that you may require some outside source (surgery, drug therapy) to accommodate.

Chronic stress accounts for a condition called *Vital Exhaustion*, which is characterized by heightened irritability, unusual tiredness, a loss of physical and mental energy, and demoralized feelings.[2] It's an indicator of chronic mental stress, which reflects a decrease in stress coping mechanisms that may contribute to an increased risk of early atherosclerosis in young healthy adults.[3] This condition is one of the key causes of coronary artery disease and subsequent heart attack.

So, substituting one stress (good) for the other (bad) is vital in creating the right atmosphere for success, removing the barriers that hinder you from walking the path that leads to your victory.

Chapter 3

ALL YOU NEED TO SUCCEED IS YOU

A s you begin your journey to wholeness and health, it will be critical for you to recognize and believe that you already have everything that you will need to succeed within. Your mind is ready to believe in victory. Your spirit is just waiting to motivate you to victorious action, and your body has the power to stay the course to victory. But until you really know that...until you act like the winner you are, the journey will not be successful

The Power of the Mind

The power of the mind to believe in victory can be seen in this story about an American hero. Wilma Rudolph was born into poverty in the state of Tennessee. When she was four years old, she contracted polio, along with suffering from a case of double pneumonia, which left her paralyzed in her left leg. She had to wear a brace in order to walk upright, and her doctor told her mother that she would *never* be able to walk normally again. Wilma must have had a praying mother, because she encouraged Wilma despite the doctor's beliefs, telling her that she could do anything she wanted to do if she only believed. Wilma had one response for the nonbelievers and naysayers: "I want to be the fastest woman on this earth."

She was prescribed to wear the brace from the moment she got out of bed until the time she went to sleep at night. She hated it. She saw it as a visible sign that she had a physical problem that separated her from everyone else, making her an outcast. Like any child, she wanted to be accepted and to fit in—be like everyone else. When her parents were not around, Wilma often took the brace off, trying to walk without a limp. She finally mastered walking, controlling her tendency to quick step on her weaker leg. In her autobiography, Wilma wrote that even as a child she was aware that "...people were going to start separating me from that brace, start thinking about me differently, start saying that Wilma is a healthy kid, just like all the rest of them."

As if that wasn't enough, Wilma grew up in the South during a time of racism and prejudice. She witnessed the glaring disparity in America's treatment of African Americans, and it made her angry and bitter. Her anger about society's treatment of African Americans would be tempered only by her Christian beliefs, which taught tolerance and forgiveness. Later she would be quoted as saying that, "she courageously [forgave] them as Christ was in her heart."

By the age of thirteen, she participated in her first race in which she came in dead last. But that didn't stop Wilma. She continued to compete, participating in countless other races until one day she broke through, taking first place. At fifteen, Wilma visited Tennessee State University where she met a coach with whom she shared her vision of becoming the fastest woman in the world. The coach must have also shared God's vision of prophetic thinking, telling her, "with your spirit nobody can stop you."

Over the years, Wilma continued to race, coming in first place through high school and college until finally, in the 1960 Olympics, Wilma Rudolph attained her goal. The once paralytic girl, who was told she would never walk normally again, became the fastest woman on earth by winning three gold medals—in the individual 100 and 200 meter run, and 4x100 meter relay.[1]

Who would have ever believed that a paralytic girl with such circumstances could have accomplished what she did? *Wilma believed in something greater than what she saw in the mirror.* That little girl that wore a brace was only the outside shell. What lived inside of her was something greater. Her perspective is what gave her hope. Wilma Rudolph may have visually seen herself as a victim, but she dreamed to live as a winner. Imagine what you could do today if you envisioned yourself the same way that Wilma Rudolph did. Some call it intestinal fortitude. But you should recognize it as the living, breathing Holy Spirit. You can tap into the potential that dwells within and dare to chase your dreams. You have that potential within you! All you need to do is believe and take the necessary steps toward victory just like Wilma did.

COSBY'S CORNER
Kitten Biscuits

Once while traveling and listening to the radio, I heard an old preacher tell a story with a powerful message—one that resonated with me about the power of finding your true identity beyond your circumstances.

There once was a female kitten that kept coming around the house, hanging around on the preacher's front porch. She was fearless, taking every opportunity to drag herself along people's legs as they entered and exited the house through the front porch. The preacher said he got really frustrated with the cat when she got tangled between his feet and almost tripped him.

Right when he was about to retaliate, he noticed that she was pregnant, and figured that all she was doing was soliciting him for food. He began to feed her twice a day, placing a small bowl of scraps and cat food just off the back porch in the grass to eliminate the annoying behavior.

This went on for a couple of weeks and then the preacher noticed that the cat had all of a sudden disappeared. He waited a couple of days for her to return, but to his surprise, nothing. He was confounded. He decided that she must have found some other place to set up camp in preparation for the delivery of her babies and moved on. A bit teary-eyed, the preacher returned back to laboring with his daily house chores and planned to remove an old stove he had in his backyard. Right when he was about to haul it away, something told him to open the door of the stove. Lo and behold, the female cat had moved into the stove and had a full litter of kittens. Witnessing this gave the preacher inspiration for a sermon the following Sunday morning; he spoke on identity in God and the importance of seeing oneself as being greater than the sum of your circumstances. He said, "I had a cat that delivered a litter of kittens inside an old stove, but that didn't make them biscuits."

Hopefully you got that. My point of the story? You can be living out a history of lies, names people called you and negative things they told you about being a failure and never amounting to anything. You could also be dealing with your own frustrations of past failures, especially weight loss, but let the past be the past.

Finally decide that you are greater than the sum of your results thus far. Stand up today and identify yourself as much more than a conqueror. You already have the victory, already won the fight. Your path of triumph is laid before you. All you have to do is decide that you can and will be something more than even you yourself have imagined you could be.

Those kittens knew they weren't biscuits, and you don't have to be the names you've been called either. (Well, you are what you eat. Sorry, couldn't pass that one up. This is a health book, you know. By the way, pass up the white flour biscuits for whole wheat, or just pass on biscuits altogether until you get where you want to be.) I'm just saying . . .

■■■

His Spirit Within Brings Success

Some of the most powerful and effective moments of my life that deal with building my relationship with the Almighty come from my acceptance that apart from Him I can do nothing. It's a rather difficult pill to swallow for most of us. I like to think that I'm truly turning things over to Him (giving Him the wheel and letting Him drive), but as time goes by and things don't seem to move at the right speed and direction that I'd like them to, I suddenly find myself grabbing the wheel and ultimately spinning out of control. It takes my surrender to the helplessness of my own humanity and diligent trust to get me back on the path.

> We are able to overcome anything that stands against us because what is inside us is greater than what is in the world.

God cautions us to remember that His dwelling place is inside of us. In 1 Corinthians 3:16 it says, "Do you not know that you are the temple of God, and that the Spirit of God dwells in you?" This is God reaching out to us, expressing that the Holy Spirit has taken sanctuary in us, that these fragile, flesh-covered skeletons have become the ultimate spiritual temple. Therefore, we are no longer slaves to this world and the temptations that exist. We are able to overcome anything that stands against us because what is inside us is greater than what is in the world.

Our thoughts will dictate the state of our hearts. If our thoughts are pure, our hearts will be pure, brimming only with the ability to overcome the deceitful, wicked traps and snares of the enemy. I love what is written in Ezekiel 36:26–27:

> Also, I will give you a new heart, and a new spirit I will
> put within you. And I will take away the stony heart
> out of your flesh, and I will give you a heart of flesh. I
> will put My Spirit within you and cause you to walk in
> My statutes.

Recall that you have just embarked on a new season in your life through God's calling. That includes having a new heart, spiritually and physically. The change you make today is instantaneous. Your heart will begin to receive a healing as soon as you determine that it is necessary. Allow God to do what He promised He would do by removing that heart of stone and replacing it with a heart of flesh. Once you do, He will pour His Spirit inside of it, and it will move you—move you into the reaping of joy and happiness that only comes from the seeds that you scatter into the world through faith and diligence. Your steadfast approach to taking back your health is not your struggle only, but one that will be fought alongside the presence of a living Savior. Stand in agreement with the idea that everything you need is right inside of you. I've given you the tools, now work in truth.

Building Your Body's Health IQ

All right, so I've been really trying to convince you that this healthier *you* thing is right at your fingertips. I've stated that we all are spirit beings who live in a body and have a soul, and that it is essential to address all three aspects if we are to truly appreciate the potential that God has for us. I firmly believe that you have the power, ability, and opportunity dwelling right inside of you. But you must become empowered by one thing: *knowledge.*

On this journey, my goal is to educate you by building up your health IQ (Individual Quota—where you want to be). This can only be done by comprehending your personal numbers. Things like blood pressure, cholesterol levels, blood sugar baselines, weight, and BMI are very important. They let you know exactly where you are compared to the healthy population. So what is healthy? What does it mean to be fit? And furthermore, what is wellness? Let me help you to know the differences between the three. Some of it may seem like a matter of semantics, but I consider it to be more of a mind-set. Let's take a look at the definitions of each one, and then I'll break it down for you.

1. **Health:** The World Health Organization defines it as "a state of complete physical, mental, and social well-being and not merely the absence of disease or infirmity."[2]

2. **Wellness:** Merriam-Webster says it is "the quality or state of being healthy."[3]

3. **Fitness:** The capability of the body to distribute inhaled oxygen to muscle tissue during increased physical effort. The President's Council on Physical Fitness and Sports does not offer a simple definition of physical fitness, but instead offers a chart that breaks it down into categories and subsets, which capture how well the body is functioning based on skill, health, and sport.[4]

Confused yet? I thought you might be. It's kind of hard to interpret the differences between the three, especially since the definitions are somewhat ambiguous. Overall, I'd summarize it as this:

> The ideal behind being healthy, having some degree of wellness, and performing at a fit level seem to be related to the efficiency of the body, mind, and spirit to operate at an optimal level. This reduces the unnecessary strain and stress on the other systems of the body, which allows the individual to achieve maximal outcomes during the normal activities of life.

Who wants to be out of breath during a quiet stroll in the park or at the shopping mall? In a nutshell, people have to *feel* good about how well they interact with their environment on a daily basis, and have confidence in how efficient their bodies are at handling stress, minus undesirable outcomes such as colds or acute illness.

Understanding Your Body's STATS

I'm going to make it easier for you. I came up with the acronym STATS. Each letter stands for a category that will help you to be in proper alignment with all three above definitions. Knowing your STATS will help better your chances of staying above the curve and operating within the fitness norms, which in turn will improve your overall health and general wellness. So let's take a look at the first one.

S: Sex

Men are from Mars and women are from Venus, right? Enough said! But consider this: there are some very pertinent differences between men and women when it comes down to health concerns, especially when speaking about the developmental cycle through the life span. Did you know that women are more likely to suffer from osteoporosis than men? As many as half of all women and a quarter of men over the age of fifty will break a bone due to osteoporosis.[5]

As pertaining to gender differences related to weight loss and exercise, men generally respond better to weight-loss effects of regular exercise.[6] This has to do mainly with the differences in body fat distribution between the sexes. It is normally stored in the upper body of males and makes for preferential fat mobilization for energy during exercise.[7] So I know this can be disconcerting for the ladies, but it just means that you will have to be that much more exacting with your dietary intake as to eliminate the ingestion of excessive amounts of fats. Men could get away with cheating a little more, but keep in mind that this will only slow your progression.

T: Total cholesterol count

Along with reading this book, I highly recommend that you first consult with your physician about having a general physical so he/she can assess your cholesterol levels. Your cholesterol is primarily synthesized from simpler substances within the body. It is required to build and maintain membranes; it modulates membranes' fluidity over the range of physiological temperatures. Cholesterol also functions in intracellular transport, cell signaling, nerve conduction, cell signaling processes, and is a precursor molecule for the synthesis of vitamin D, steroid hormones, and sex hormones progesterone, estrogens, and testosterone.

In other words, you need cholesterol. But beyond what the body normally synthesizes, we put a lot of excess cholesterol in our bodies through our dietary intake. Watching what we consume can drastically improve our cholesterol values. Be aware that there is good (HDL) and bad (LDL) cholesterol. I will not bore you with any more details, but I will give you some norms to look for. *See following chart*:

Level mg/dL	Level mmol/L	Interpretation
< 200	< 5.2	Desirable level corresponding to lower risk for heart disease
200–240	5.2–6.2	Borderline high risk
> 240	> 6.2	High risk

A: Activity level

How about this one? How important is your energy or activity level as pertaining to wellness, or more specifically, fitness? More significant than you know! I'll tell you why. It all has to do with a process called *homeostasis*. Defined, it's the property of a system that regulates its internal environment and tends to maintain a stable, constant condition of properties like temperature or pH. The human body manages a multitude of highly complex interactions on a daily basis in order to maintain balance or to return systems to functioning within a normal range (example: heart and respiratory rate). These interactions within the body facilitate compensatory changes supportive of physical and psychological functioning, which is essential to the survival of the individual or species. Failure to do so causes shutdown, mutation, or even sudden death—none of which is an attractive option. How does the body do it? Through another important process called *metabolism*. I know, I know. Everybody hates that word because it infers that the average three-hundred-pound person who has a lineage of overweight or obesity running in the family doesn't have a snowball's chance in you know where to lose as much weight as the average one-hundred-fifty pounder. Well, sit back and read as I break it down a little for you and shed some light on this otherwise dark truth.

Webster has two definitions for *metabolism*:

1. The sum of the processes in the buildup and destruction of protoplasm; specifically: the chemical changes in living cells by which energy is provided for vital processes and activities and new material is assimilated.[8]

2. The sum of the processes by which a particular substance is handled in the living body.[9]

In other words, the sum total of the chemical reactions that go on in living cells, which allows for reactions by which the body obtains and spends the energy from food, is energy metabolism. At least two-thirds of the energy the average person spends in a day supports the body's metabolic activity. Therefore, it's just a measure of how well our bodies complete chemical reactions to release energy for use or storage (when too much energy is available and not needed). The last part is the problem. Did you know that fat is nothing more than stored energy? Your body is smart, people. It stores away what it does not need right now.

> Performing exercises that use more muscle groups simultaneously will produce greater energy expenditures, thus speeding up the body's need to produce more muscle mass, which in turn produces more energy.

So this is great news, right? You no longer have to

be intimidated by metabolism. Still confused? Let's look at metabolism just a little bit closer. During digestion, the body breaks down three energy yielding nutrients—carbohydrates, lipids, and proteins—into four units that can be absorbed into the blood: glucose, glycerol, fatty acids, and amino acids. All of these nutrients are used to build muscle, repair injured cells, build new cells, and so much more. In other words, YOU NEED THEM! But just not the amount that you normally consume; metabolism is measured by your basal metabolic rate (BMR)—the rate of energy used for metabolism under basal (normal) conditions.

Factors that affect BMR are age, height, growth, body composition, hormones, caffeine, sleep, stresses, and environmental temperature. Some of these things you just can't change. But, BMR can be manipulated by the activity level related to energy output. Activity causes an expenditure of energy, which

> Just because you hang out in the gym for two to three hours at a time does not guarantee you will lose that spare tire or those love handles.

forces the body to use more nutrients to fuel functions such as movement, delivery of oxygen via the heart and lungs, and disposal of wastes. The amount of energy needed is dependent on three things: *muscle mass, body weight, and the activity.*

Take home tip: the larger the muscle mass required and the heavier the weight of the body part to be moved, the more energy is spent. So, the three-hundred-pound person from earlier can expend more energy per workout than the one-hundred-fifty pound person. What needs to be done in order to achieve this is to select the right exercise prescription based on the goals for each individual. Performing exercises that use more muscle groups simultaneously will produce greater energy expenditures, thus speeding up the body's need to produce more muscle mass, which in turn produces more energy. And the cycle goes on and on over time. Running, skiing, and even playing basketball expend more energy than aerobics and walking.

T: Training regimen

You may ask the question, "What is a good training regimen? I challenge you to instead ask the question: "What kind of regimen is right *for me*?" Here's why: it's a fact that most exercise programs aim at meeting goals such as losing weight, building more muscle, and increasing activity tolerance—all the wrong angles. The reason these goals are wrong is because they try to place people in programs that work well for others, rather than structuring programs that work

> It's simple: if you want big arms, legs, chest, and back muscles—lift big. If you want lean, flexible, and strong arms, waist, legs, and hips—do cardio exercises and lift moderate weight.

well for that individual. Working along the right parameters that meet both the expectations and goals of the individual and utilize that person's strengths, while accounting for their weaknesses, is much more effective and productive. Most people go to the gym and work out like crazy, spending countless hours there, which, quite honestly, wastes a lot of time. Just because you hang out in the gym for two to three hours at a time does not guarantee you will lose that spare tire or those love handles. You have to first make goals for yourself that include each body part you want to improve, and then perform the appropriate exercises that target those areas. It's an exercise principle called *specificity of exercise.*

It's simple: if you want big arms, legs, chest, and back muscles—lift big. If you want lean, flexible, and strong arms, waist, legs, and hips—do cardio exercises and lift moderate weight. Example: volleyball players don't really emphasize bench press and pushups because they need to be flexible in that area so they can open their chest and hit the ball over the net. Therefore, they focus on back muscles and pectoral muscle flexibility. Another example: take the average NFL offensive lineman. He plays a full NFL football game, and each play lasts for about three to five seconds. He needs to be able to perform at a high rate for only three to five seconds, then take a rest break. It would be insane for him to train like a marathon runner because it is unnecessary for the skill of his profession.

It is the same for those of us trying to meet our personal fitness and wellness goals. *Want to lose weight?* Increase the number of calories burned per day and decrease those consumed. *Want to put on more muscle?* Lift heavy weights and provide the body

> Customize your program to cater to your own personal strengths and weaknesses.

with foods such as protein and carbohydrates so that the body can adapt to the stress by building more muscle. *Want to lean-up, especially around the hips and waist?* Cardio, plus strength training, along with a healthy diet that encourages high energy foods loaded with fiber and protein, will help you to increase metabolism.

The great thing about working out is that there are so many different types of exercise programs that you can participate in. That way, you are in full control of your own dedication to the right plan that will help you to accomplish your goals. Boot camps, Chachersize, Bollywood, salsa dancing, free weights, circuit training, Zumba, and water aerobics are just a few that fit a person in a specific way that addresses that person's overall fitness. You can customize your program to cater to your own personal strengths and weaknesses.

Now the sad part is that it just isn't that simple. You may have tried and tested many of these routines without success. But don't give up! That's why you're reading this book, right? With persistent customization, along with trial and error, you can catalogue your successes and failures and identify the modified regimen that's right for you.

S: Spiritual alignment

Here's where we talk about the importance of the spiritual connection between setting your personal goals and walking in the power of God and His will and purpose for your life. You need to align yourself with what He has planned for you, and tapping into the scriptures for encouragement and building that aforementioned relationship is the only way. I already touched on this in the spirit section of this chapter.

All right, so I just made you smarter, right? Of course I did, because think about it, you just learned more about your body in a matter of minutes than you could glean burning a few hours perusing the Internet or thumbing through a book. I simplified the process for you. And so, now here's the million dollar question: What are you going to do with all that knowledge? Well, I'll tell you. You're going to get serious about it. Those STATS are going to be the compass to navigate you through the jungle of unhealthiness. Consider it to be the framework for your fitness survival kit. With it you will be able to gauge how healthy you really are—or at least how much healthier you are becoming. Conceptualize it like this: as you implement your new training regimen, you will begin to lose weight and that will drop your BMI, which will in turn increase your activity level, dropping your cholesterol back into normal ranges. All of this will go a long way to keeping you motivated and working even harder to get greater results. Along the way, don't forget to sharpen up that spiritual alignment. Rome wasn't built in a day and in those tough times when you just don't feel like doing anything, only strength from a higher power will carry you through.

Chapter 4

SINS OF THE FATHER

N O ONE EXISTS as an island unto himself. In this chapter we will discover the foundation for health that has been established already by the influences of the people and cultures from which we come. This is a very interesting chapter to me, because it speaks to a special place in my heart that I honestly believe everyone shares. Your foundation for eating begins in this place, and throughout your life span, many additional things will play a role in shaping what kind of eater you will be.

Our parents are the ones responsible for setting things in motion. We were born, vulnerable to the world, and our primary requirement from them was food. We cried, and our parents mercifully obliged us. Early on they provided milk, then they started to introduce more solid foods, and so ultimately we were able to eat full meals. During this early process, our internal schedules and the condition of our stomachs were set at a somewhat stationary state.

The Desire of the Mind to Be Satiated

By the time our stomachs had adjusted to a certain amount of food that we needed to receive to be satiated, our parents had subconsciously installed two components of our eating habits: an internal time-clock and an internal measuring cup. This created a habitual eating pattern in both our mind and our body that, for the most part, is still with many of us to this day.

Along with that, we have the cultural and socioeconomic norms that dictate how we eat. Depending on your class background—upper, middle, lower class—the availability of food plays a major role in the quantity and quality of food. Culturally, the type and amount of food consumed is relevant. Some cultures eat foods that are high in starch, carbohydrates, calories, and cholesterol, while others follow diets that are rich in a balance of the vegetables, lean meats, fish, and whole grains. You don't have to be a medical professional to predict the negative impact this plays on the general health of our cardiovascular, neurological, digestive, and musculoskeletal systems.

> Our foundation for health has been established by the influences of the people and cultures from which we come.

If you assess your familial history and account for the present state of your own health right now, I'm sure there is a direct correlation between the things I just spoke of and where you are right now. If you're in the negative, you have my sympathy. Your focus of control during this time of your life was minimal, and therefore, out of your control. I call these *the sands of our fathers*. But you know how the saying goes: "It isn't where you came from; it's where you're going that counts,"[1] and today you have a chance to make a change."

"Finish Your Plate!"

I know personally for me, one of the big things that affected my eating habits was something that my mother and my grandmother always emphasized. They told me to finish my plate. Most times it always came down to the vegetables. I hated them. I pushed them onto the side and finished everything else on my plate until finally, staring me in the face was a pile of vegetables I had avoided all night. So there I sat, hopelessly waiting for some miraculous event to come along and wash those veggies away. But it never came.

My grandmother and mother did everything to convince me. They threatened that I wouldn't be able to look at TV if I didn't finish. They told me that I could not get dessert if I didn't finish. They even went as far as telling me that I would not be able to eat dinner the next day until I finished eating my vegetables from the night before. Thank God that none of that ever had to happen to convince me, but you can see how powerful this could have been to my psyche.

On the positive side, they were teaching me the value of eating vegetables; I give them credit for that. But there were some nights when vegetables were not the last thing on my plate, and they still pushed the ideal that I needed to clean my plate. They told me those familiar

> I found myself finishing my plate no matter how big or little it was.

stories we've all heard at one time or another—about starving children all over the world, and homeless kids in the United

States, and how I should be appreciative that I had a meal placed before me.

Not a bad idea by any means; I'm not knocking them on that. But what they taught me as a child ultimately followed me into my adulthood. I found myself finishing my plate no matter how big or little it was. Something inside me needled at the back of my mind until it drilled through my brain, landing at a place right behind my eyeballs, convincing me that if I didn't finish my plate I had committed some unforgivable sin. I had no choice but to follow through. I was brainwashed!

> Eating has become a rote activity that many of us do without even getting to the point of being hungry.

I was fortunate enough to be an active child, so all those extra calories went to a good place, giving me the necessary energy to get through my day without storing any extra calories as fat.

So much of what we eat, when we eat, and how we eat is mental. We don't even think about it. Eating has become a rote activity that many of us do without even getting to the point of being hungry. You don't believe me? What about that kid who always wants to eat when he sees someone else with food? It's probably no surprise to find that that same child has become a social eater who takes samples from other folks' plates when at a gathering. He probably isn't even hungry. He sees food and has to eat because no one stopped this habit at the root. My grandmother used to say, "Monkey see; monkey do."

Do you consider yourself a social eater? If you do, ask your parents what kind of kid you were. I'm willing to wager that you acted in a similar fashion way back then. But you have freedom now. You can look in the mirror and tell yourself that you are going to try to start training your body to eat only when you need to eat. You will no longer be a slave to the intrinsic practices of your childhood. You will take control and master your desires, developing a stronger eating conscience to cultivate a lifestyle more beneficial to not just you, but your family as well. Those things that your parents, culture, and socioeconomic circumstances imparted on you will no longer be a stronghold in your life. You will walk in the freedom that God has given you.

COSBY'S CORNER
Which came first,
the fried chicken or the egg?

Interesting question, right? I just wanted to catch your attention, if I hadn't already done so. Let's rephrase it to, What to eat: fried chicken or eggs? The answer is obvious that it should be eggs, silly. At least I hope you answered eggs.

I wanted to take a short break to talk about the health benefits of eggs. Eggs are underrated. Eggs are great for the eyes in two ways: they help prevent macular degeneration due to lutein and zeaxanthin. These nutrients are more readily available to be used by our bodies than any other substance. Also, people who eat eggs every day are at lower risk of developing cataracts.

Another reason to eat eggs: protein power! One egg contains six grams of high-quality protein and all nine essential amino acids (building blocks of protein). One egg yolk has about 300mcg of choline, which is an important nutrient that helps regulate the brain, nervous system, and cardiovascular system.

Here's a good one: eggs may also help to prevent breast cancer. In one study, women who consumed at least six eggs per week lowered their risk of breast cancer by 44 percent.[2]

Last point, eggs are one of the only foods that contain naturally occurring vitamin D, which is great for developing strong bones, immune system regulation, and maintain body weight.

Now for the benefits of fried chicken. Give me a minute here to look through my notes...

Oh, sorry, I don't have any data collected as of yet. But I'm sure someone out there in cyberspace has something good to say. Feel free to look there because you will not find it here.

I love chicken, just not fried. I used to be a fried chicken fool though. My favorite fast food fried chicken place had me hooked like an addict. Every week, they'd see my face, asking for the family special with spicy chicken on the bottom and mild on top. Yep, that's how I remember it.

But alas, I just became too educated to keep exposing myself to the vast amounts of saturated fat, trans fats, and any other fat that exists. The clogging of my arteries became so unfashionable, a trend best left to those who don't mind having high blood pressure and possibly suffering a heart attack or stroke anytime in the near future.

Look, don't get upset at me for saying it, because someone has to. You are what you eat, it's true. You can either become a person with ideal body weight, great vision, strong bones, great immune and cardiovascular systems, and at a lower risk of developing certain forms of cancer. Or you can just settle for being someone who is overweight, with high blood pressure, and a BMI that gives you a higher probability of having a heart attack or stroke. I'm just saying...

■■■

Our Spirit Is Designed to Be Free

Spiritually, the Bible speaks about the freedom that God has given us. And not just over food, but over everything in our lives. We have the freedom of choice, we have the freedom of discernment, and we even have freedom from the iniquity of our parents, habits, addictions, and behavior. Some of these things are of a spiritual nature, passed down from generation to generation. Exodus 20:5 touches on this: "...visiting the iniquity of the fathers on the children to the third and fourth generation."

These offenses are unfairly passed down to us, and we unknowingly walk in them until we medically present with the same diseases and disabilities. It's labeled as *heredity*, but I'd like to look at it through spiritual lenses, seeing it for what it truly is: *spiritual curses*.

Even Solomon in all his manifold wisdom fell into this spiritual trap. His father King David faltered before God while coveting Bathsheba. He did whatever he inclined his heart to do to have her, even plotting to kill her husband. That desire to have a woman rested on Solomon. During his reign as king, he had seven hundred wives and three hundred

> God can save us from our family iniquities. We no longer have to be victims.

concubines. In 1 Kings 15:3 we see that King David's other son Abijah became king of Judah. During his three year reign it says that: "He walked in all the sins of his father that he had done before him."

Spiritual curses are by no means a respecter of persons. From kings to peasants, no one is safe and everyone can fall victim to them. We have to be grounded in the foundation that God can save us from our family iniquities. We no longer have to be victims. God identified the trend of sin and the curses that encompassed our lineage, and graciously released us from these snares. In Ezekiel 18:20, God states, "The soul who sins shall die. The son shall not bear the punishment of the iniquity of the father, nor shall the father bear the punishment of the iniquity of the son." We will no longer be riddled with the sin and guilt of our parents. God has willfully declared that we can operate in our own free will. Only the things that we decide to do will be counted against us. Therefore, you can receive this liberty with thanksgiving. Starting right now, decide that nothing will hold you back from achieving success. It is your spiritual inheritance to do so, given to you freely by God Almighty.

Spiritual Foundations Influence Your Body

Let's consider the power of the spiritual foundations established by our parents and culture as relating to the diseases of excess weight. Here is my list of the top ten co-morbidities that accompany obesity:

1. Type II diabetes

2. Depression

3. Pulmonary complications (obstructive sleep apnea, pulmonary hypertension)

4. Liver disease (not associated with alcohol)

5. Some forms of cancer

6. Cardiovascular disease (stroke, myocardial infarction [heart attack], atrial fibrillation)

7. Metabolic syndrome (hypercholesterolemia, hypertension)

8. Acute pancreatitis

9. Gallbladder disease

10. Osteoarthritis[3]

The cultural disparities of obesity in America are frightening. A study performed in 2007–2008 produced these results concerning obesity percentages amongst the population.[4]

• Non-hispanic whites, 32.8 percent

• Non-hispanic blacks, 44.1 percent

• All hispanics, 37.9 percent

• Mexican American, 39.3 percent

A report in 2010 by the National Center for Health Statistics supports the daunting correlation between socioeconomic status and obesity. The results are no less alarming than the study above.[5]

- 33 percent of men who live in households with low income level (below the poverty line) are obese, while 29.2 percent of men who live above the poverty level are obese.

- 29.0 percent of women who live in households with low income level (below the poverty line) are obese, while 42.0 percent of women who live above the poverty level are obese.

In summary, the staggering association between obesity and either culture or socioeconomic status paints a clear picture for you as to the predictability of obesity. Hopefully, where you may have been discouraged or worried about this type of data, you should feel empowered. You no longer have to follow in the same traditions of old that have predestined you to sickness and disease. In Hosea 4:6 God says, "My people are destroyed for lack of knowledge." I have provided that knowledge to you. Now use it to galvanize that inner desire that I *know* lives in you to become a healthier person going forward, breaking away from those sins.

Chapter 5

TURN DOWN THE VOLUME AND LISTEN

I N THIS CHAPTER I want you to come to grips with this truth: there is no magic pill that exists to get the weight off and turn you into an overnight success at weight loss! People love to think they can just dictate the rate at which they lose weight, but I'm willing to bet that the vast majority of people who finally decide to get serious about weight loss have come to grips with this reality: If it's done the right way, it's going to take time. There is no diet program or exercise video or routine that will shed layers of fat from your body overnight.

Wrap Your Mind Around the Issue of Volume

If you want to get amazing results, you will have to attack weight loss on two fronts—eating volume and exercise. I don't care how hard you work or starve yourself (which is actually counterproductive to weight loss), it will not budge. Remember, you most likely put those pounds on through years of hard work and dedication to the cause of feeding yourself. Now it's time to commit to the hard work and time of learning to manage the volume issue—meaning to manage your portion size, cut back on calorie consumption, and put in the time of intense workouts at the gym. Here's one easy rule to remember: if it's bigger than your fist, don't put it in your mouth.

> If you want to get amazing results, you will have to attack weight loss on two fronts—eating volume and exercise.

Wrap your mind around the knowledge that it is going to take discipline and self-control on your part to strip off that excess weight from your musculoskeletal frame. Oh yeah, you have one of those. It's just hiding underneath all that...what I'll kindly call that stored, unused energy.

Let's face the truth: if you want to lose weight, serious weight, you're going to have to attack the eating and the exercise components with equal amounts of conviction. No one way is better or more essential than the other. But the good news for you is that once you learn how to do it, it will indeed yield the results you've been dreaming of.

This chapter is going to make you think smarter about what you have been doing to your body and what you will do to your body from now on to make it a calorie-crunching, energy-producing, metabolism-ramping, and fat-burning machine.

My friend Jamie Dukes is a living testimony of someone who made the switch and has lost more than 100 pounds. He did, however, need a little push to get him going first. That push came in the form of a surgical intervention.

Back in 2009, Jamie said he wanted, no *needed*, to make a change in his life. Jamie is a retired NFL player who watched four ex-teammates of his die from complications and diseases of excess weight. Jamie was an offensive lineman for four NFL teams over the span of a ten-year career. He needed to maintain a certain body mass in order to be competitive enough to turn back crashing opposing team defenders during each contest. Lifting weights four hours a day and eating to replenish energy stores and build muscle was the routine that helped him meet the criteria. But by the time Jamie was at the end of his career, his last playing weight hung around 305 pounds.

After his retirement from the NFL, Jamie no longer had the same regimen of daily exercise. Along with that, his hectic work schedule made it difficult to control what he was consuming on the road. As time went on, Jamie's weight increased to around 405 pounds, putting him at risk of suffering a heart attack or stroke. He battled with high blood pressure and elevated cholesterol levels, things that are the recipe for cooking up a successful life-ending tragedy. "All the weight loss and diet programs I tried weren't working," Jamie said. He realized he needed something to get the needle on the scale moving in the right direction. He wanted a *jump start* to making a life change and decided to undergo the surgical intervention of lap-band surgery (a band placed around the stomach that makes it smaller).

Jamie's physician said that Jamie was exercising and making decent food choices, but he was losing the battle against *volume*. The band allowed Jamie to eat the food he wanted, but in lower portions. Jamie now had the extra push he needed. With the

> Understand the importance of attacking weight management the right way.

volume consumption piece in place, Jamie was able to focus on increasing the amount of exercise, and, over time, Jamie was able to cut down the weight drastically. Now, Jamie weighs in at two hundred eighty-five pounds and is exercising three to four times a week minimum.

I shared this with you not so that you would go out and seek out a bariatric surgeon, but so that you can understand the importance of attacking weight management the right way. It's going to take a strong will and an ironclad heart of determination to do it. But I know you can. You just have to make up your mind. The good news is you already have.

COSBY'S CORNER
Fat Ways

NFL analyst Jamie D. Dukes and I first started the radio show *Ask the Fat Doctors* as a podcast, and one night his wife, Angela, joined us on the show. Needless to say, when the lady of the house speaks, it's best to just sit back and listen. Beyond just the hot topics and social media highlights, Angela shared with us something that I thought was an amazing observation. She said that people have problems with weight loss because they develop what she calls "fat ways." She made it up, I cosigned it—well, really stole it—and now I'm going to share it with you.

Imagine this. One Friday night you're all alone in the house, and your favorite interval of television shows is about to come on over the next two hours. Or maybe it's your favorite movie you pop into the DVD player. Anyway, you settle in for the night, and decide that there is only one thing that can make this moment even better—a bowl of your favorite ice cream! You go to the freezer, pull the ice cream carton out, and grab a bowl. Right before you grab the ice cream scooper, you say to yourself, "Wait a minute. I'm the only one who eats this kind of ice cream. So why do I need to use a bowl? I will just take it with me and eat a little bit right out of the box."

Before you know it, what you intended to be only a few more spoonfuls turns into half the carton, and then matriculates into the entire box of ice cream being devoured. What's that spell? Fat way!

Are you guilty of this behavior? It is the type of thing that will keep you overweight and on the path of life change destruction. I can hear you now: "That's not me. I never eat the entire carton." OK, a fat way is not just limited to only ice cream. What about the entire bag of potato chips or the whole bag of powdered doughnuts?

Let's try this one: I go into my cabinet and latch on to the bag of cookies, take a tall glass of milk, and get to some serious dunking. "Oh no, I ate the whole bag." Fat ways! I've been there before, trust me on that one.

Are you the type to take the two-liter soda bottle with you, or better yet, the pizza box? Please take the time to write down your fat way and leave it right next to the note that I asked you to make earlier with your goals written on it. Make sure it is posted in the same area that is supposed to stop you from losing out.

Scary thing is, you may have more than just one fat way. But be strong, first identify each one, and then remove them one by one. Remember what the moral of the above testimony is, people: VOLUME CONTROL! Not as in the sound of me screaming at you, but more like the sights and sounds of you eating. You did it, not me. I'm just saying...

■■■

Find Your Spiritual Balance

I'm going to break away from just food talk here to touch on the importance of having spiritual balance in order to truly free yourself from the clutches of the evil excess weight pitfall. In the Bible, God speaks about spiritual fruit. It is important to understand the concept of tapping into the spiritual aspect of health and wellness if you are to truly empower yourself to break past cycles of defeat. I think people develop inward scars that manifest into outward lesions, and the cycle self-propagates until they are overwhelmed by an overpowering whirlwind of emotion. The cycles of love and hate, anger and frustration, eventually create invisible walls at the subconscious level that drive people to eat in order to feel better about their circumstances. This isn't true of everyone who is overweight. But, we have to admit that we are human beings whose actions and reactions are often driven by intense emotions from within.

> It is important to understand the concept of tapping into the spiritual aspect of health and wellness if you are to truly empower yourself to break past cycles of defeat.

Our free will is all that most of us have left, and even some of that has been stripped away from us through our low sense of self-worth based on past experiences and relationships. Food is a good substitute for many things. The sugar rushes that lift our spirits on a dreary day and the release of more than three hundred chemicals when we consume chocolate have varied effects on the nervous system. So we can't ignore the natural tendency to eat when our emotions are out of whack.

I know that when I am bored, I eat. Don't know why I do it, but I can't help myself. If I am home alone and don't have anything to do with myself, I will travel to the refrigerator over and over again, open the door and look inside. Sometimes, I open it multiple times within the hour, not finding anything to eat, and then returning as if I missed something or like someone put food in there when I wasn't looking.

God has the answer to our troubled minds—the fruits of the Spirit. In Paul's letter to the Galatians, he addresses this topic in chapter 5 verses 22–23:

> But the fruit of the Spirit is love, joy, peace, patience, gentleness, goodness, faith, meekness, and self-control; against such there is no law.

Paul says that these are the fruits of the Spirit. Therefore one would assume that you have to have already tapped into the Holy Spirit in order to reap the fruits of the Spirit. You must accept the fact that the presence of the Holy Spirit dwells in you and is present around you. It is not just some mystical ideal that some people are able to press into and unveil signs of miracles and wonders. It is something that God sent to man as a gift and a promise.

The *Comforter* that Jesus Himself promised to send in the Gospels before He ascended back to heaven is very present now. You have the potential to flow in the gifts of the Spirit just as much as

> Love yourself enough to open your mind to trusting God with everything.

the great men and women of the Bible, and even the fantastic men and women of God today. God is no respecter of persons.

The best thing about it all is that you can start your first miracle by working on yourself. Get yourself right mentally, physically, and spiritually so that you can be a living testimony to others and help to advance the kingdom through your example of perseverance. Now that you accept the Spirit, you can live in His fruit. These are the things that your spirit needs to keep your soul at peace. Let's break down each one.

Love

It is essential that you have love, because the Bible teaches that there is no greater thing than this. How can you love others if you do not first love yourself? You must determine that God loves you and has made you to be a wonderful person of faith to be utilized in the pathway of fulfilling His perfect will on this planet. Love yourself enough to open your mind to trusting God with everything. Once you do this, you can be used to do great works without it being tainted by motive or vain glory.

Joy

How about joy? Where are you looking for joy? Is it in some person, at work, or even with food? In Nehemiah 8:10 we read: "For the joy of the LORD is your strength." You must find the joy from communion with God and then you will possess the strength to do what is necessary to meet your goals. Need to finish that last lap around the track? Think about the joy of the Lord. Struggling to complete that last set of sit-ups? Nothing like the joy of the Lord to get you there. Put your joy in the hands of a risen Savior who wants nothing more than to fill you up with strength so that you can be the mighty warrior that He desires for you to be.

Peace

Do you have peace at night when you go to sleep? Is your mind clouded with fear, anxiety, and restlessness about the things of this world? You need to tap into and build a relationship with God that parallels that of a son or daughter to a father. Know that God does not miss anything. He sees everything that you do and think. If you are discouraged, He is able to encourage you beyond what anything or anyone can supply. To obtain the peace, you must first find the source of peace.

Forbearance

This word can be defined a few ways: "To pause, delay; to refuse; to decline; to restrain from action; to abstain from and to avoid doing."[1] Now, take any one of the definitions and apply it to the things that you struggle with. Is it your anger? Is it your tongue? Is it your thoughts? Is it your guilt? Is it sin? It is your hate? Is it coveting? Or is it your overindulgence?

Whatever the case may be, the Spirit is coaxing us to forbear. He is giving us the gift of forbearance. We no longer need to be slaves to our own behavior, thoughts, actions, motives, and circumstances. We can walk in freedom and leave those things which hinder us behind. This will give us the freedom to truly move in the direction that God is beckoning us to follow. Then and only then will we see the correct path.

Kindness/goodness

Are you really kind? Do you do the things you do for other people for reward, reputation, or honor? Or do you give from a kind and pure heart? If you do, you have the gift of kindness.

But many of us don't. It probably has more to do with a low balance in our kindness account. People haven't shown you kindness so how can you make a withdrawal and show kindness back to such a cruel and harsh world?

You can't give what you don't have, at least not in the natural world. But in the spiritual realm, there is an abundance of kindness. It flows from an account that has no end. It cannot and will not ever give you the message of insufficient funds. If you begin to be kind to others more than the world is kind to you, I promise that your Father in heaven sees what you do and will reward you above and beyond measure.

And you know what—it will be instantaneous. You will feel good about what you are doing at that very moment, and you will obtain the mental freedom you need. Then, goodness will flow freely through you. You will be overjoyed by the expression of kindness and goodness and mercy will follow you all the days of your life.

Faithfulness

I love the song "Great Is Thy Faithfulness" because it is so true. God is faithful to do all that He says He will do. However,

> Ask God to show you what He requires of you on a daily basis, and ask yourself if you are willing to be faithful in it.

some of it comes at the price of our being obedient and holding up our end of the bargain. Whether we get with the program or not, God will be regarded as faithful. The Spirit offers us the chance to walk in this gift, but we must be willing to seek out the will of God in our lives. If we know what He wants us to do—requires us to do—we can commit to it. We may fail at it, but there is no stipulation of being perfect. We must remember to attempt to do better next time. As we continually commit to the ideal, the Spirit will enable us to improve our performance over and over again until it becomes more of a habit and less of a chore.

You might be asking, "What is he talking about? Can you be more specific?" I leave that part up to you. Search your heart. Ask God to show you what He requires of you on a daily basis, and ask yourself if you are willing to be faithful in it. All God needs is your availability to be used, and He will do the rest. He will set you up for the opportunities to show your faithfulness if you truly ask Him to.

Gentleness

I like to think of this fruit as the softest thing I can imagine. I liken it to the touch on my cheeks when my daughters give me a kiss. It's the softest and sweetest thing on the planet to me. Imagine if my actions could be akin to that. What if people could experience that same warm glow inside when I did something for them? Man, I'd be handing it out free of charge. I wish everyone could feel what I feel.

But now imagine if you were to walk in such a sweet fruit that comes from the Holy Spirit. People could try to do things to you, talk about you, wish bad on you, and even attempt to convince others how bad you are, and you could just keep on moving forward, free of their attempted mockery. The gentleness of the Holy Spirit will saturate you in an impenetrable cloud so that you can give that to others, even your enemies that they too might be saved.

Self-control

Twinkie alert, Twinkie alert, hold the Twinkies please. That's what I'm talking about. Those cute little golden-brown morsels of joy that seem to satisfy any and every craving. Yes, I love them too. But I don't eat an entire box in one sitting. I know better than that. Now, you do too.

Once the Holy Spirit gifts you with this fruit, all the Twinkies in the world won't matter. They won't make a dent in your conviction to change your life. Your fitness goals will continue to be pushed to higher limits, your exercise sessions will be increased, your workouts intensified, and your confidence will soar higher than ever before because you will have self-control as your shield from the onslaught of temptation.

It's not the circumstances that are the problem, it's how you respond to them that defines who you are. But remember this: it's not who you are, but whose you are that makes the difference. You are royalty, set apart from the rest of the world. At one time, you were misled and confused, tortured by your own willingness to follow your emotions and ignore sound reason. But once the Spirit gives you the fruit of self-control, you are able to press on toward the mark of the prize that God has laid before you, and through that your goals will be reached without strain or human effort.

You are looking for a healing and supernatural experience all at the same time. How can you have such high expectations for breakthrough if you are not willing to tap into the supernatural realm? It is the place where victory dwells. It is the place where only the Holy Spirit can take you. Don't go the road alone.

The Great Body Debate: Inches Versus Pounds

It only matters to the eye of the beholder—and I mean, beholder. Look, if you continue to believe for one second that losing two inches off your waistline is more impactful than twenty pounds, I have to be honest with you. You're wrong. I'm talking to my overweight and obese folks here. Let me make it a little more real for you.

You go to the doctor for an annual physical. Your numbers are off concerning cholesterol, blood sugar, and blood pressure. He or she tells you that you need to lose weight, right? So you go and start a diet plan that should help you level off and take these numbers into the safe range. After about a month, you notice that your waistline is slimmer, but the numbers on the scale are the same. Frustrated, you blame it on the fact that you started working out and it must be the fact that you've developed more muscle, making you heavier in the absence of fat. Nice try!

Honestly, it takes a lot more working out than that to build muscle. Matter of fact, eating more calories and supplementing in a workout that focuses on building muscle is the only sure way to secure that so-called theory into law. Most of which is probably not really happening, am I right?

Good! Now that we're being honest, let's get down to business. Truth be told, muscle does weigh more than fat. But, in most cases of individuals trying to lose weight, any weight that sheds off the scale is mainly attributed to water weight. Just the fact that you change your eating habits and add in a little more activity allows at least three to five pounds of water loss from sweat and voiding alone. So, once you get that off, now you're working on the fat.

It takes thirty-five hundred calories to account for one pound of fat—adding or subtracting. So, if all else stays the same, working out in the gym to the tune of thirty-five hundred calories, and not eating anything, will allow you to lose one pound per day. Too bad you starved yourself in the process, because you may have lost even more if you added on some muscle. But since the body starved itself and was apprehensive about expending energy to create new muscle, you didn't.

So how does it work then? Best results are slow and steady, with just the right amount of cardiovascular exercise and weight lifting. That way you can tone (add on the muscle to raise your body's metabolism) and burn (taking off fat along the way). Three meals a day with two snacks in between and a healthy regimen of weight training will carve your body into shape like an experienced sculptor. Patience is key, along with constantly pushing your body to new levels each time so that you can force it to make positive changes.

> Inches lost without weight loss equals nothing!

Inches lost without weight loss equals nothing! Stop thinking muscle was substituted for fat. In some extreme cases, this may be right. But come on, let's be truthful; it's probably more pie in the sky thinking. Remember this: "'All things are lawful to me,' but not all things are helpful" (1 Cor. 6:12). Everything is permissible, *but* not everything is beneficial. Determine that you will not be mastered by anything. "Therefore glorify God in your body" (v. 20).

You can do it all (*eat bad, smoke, drink, be sedentary*), but it may not be the best for you. Do those things that will benefit you now and in the long run. A healthy body does just that.

Follow a Good Eating Regimen

Everybody has cheat sheets to offer you when it's time to get down to losing weight, so I would be remiss if I couldn't give you a little something to give you an edge in your battle of breaking those defeating cycles when it

> Take your hand and splay it out—all fingers fully extended, along with the thumb. That should be your plate size.

comes to wellness. So, I have two gifts for you in this section:

1. Seven foods that help to boost your metabolism, with three fitness builders.

2. A simple equation that makes calorie counting easy.

With these two little nuggets, you should be well on your way to managing your intake so that fat just slides from your frame with no shame. I'm going to give you the basics of eating first.

1. Use a plate that is no bigger than your open hand (includes fingers).

Let's take a closer look at your plate. How big should your plate be? Take your hand and splay it out—all fingers fully extended, along with the thumb. That should be your plate size. A simple rule of thumb that many people consider to be true is that your stomach should be equivalent to the size of your fist, give or take a few inches here or there. Though the deviations do vary among ethnicities and gender, if you eat right, there really is no need for your stomach to be super big. So I recommend eating from a plate that is no bigger than your hand full open, including fingers, so that you can guarantee that you may be stretching your stomach, but not overfilling it.

You should not want to feel full. It's not normal for your body to be in this state of shock. Yes, it's in a state of shock. Why do you think you don't feel like doing anything right after a heavy meal? It's because your body has to shunt a majority of the blood in your body to the organs of digestion in order to break down all that stuff you just ingested. Therefore, the brain, heart, and lungs are left feeling *drained*, and all you'd rather do is lie down and rest, which is the worst possible thing you could do.

The stomach is mostly constructed of muscle. There are four layers of muscle at work in the stomach. So the more you stretch a muscle by overeating, the more it is forced to lengthen over time. With each bout of stretching, you are asking your stomach to conform to the routine of being over-stretched, which in time results in a stomach that almost craves to be filled.

You eat, you fill it up, it stretches, then it empties, you eat again. If you fail to fill it up next time, what does the stomach do? It begs for food. It desires to be filled because it has been trained to do so by your consistent actions. You feel a slow churning or grumbling in your abdomen. Other than digestion taking place, your stomach is signaling that it may be time to eat.

You have the choice to make a defining decision: feed it or ignore it. Most likely you eat, but is that really the right choice? If you are seriously trying to lose weight, you are going to have to start ignoring your stomach and listen to your mind. You've already eaten, albeit a smaller portion, but you had enough food to satisfy yourself for the next three hours until either snack time or your next meal.

From now on, you are on strict doctor's orders to turn off

the part of your brain (hypothalamus) that listens to your stomach, and focus on the one (limbic system) that is determined to meet your goals. If you stop stretching your stomach, it will begin to shrink in size. You then must start to retrain your mouth and eyes to be satisfied with consuming smaller portions throughout the day as opposed to three larger meals. This guarantees a slower release of sugar into the bloodstream, which makes you feel more satisfied longer. When it is time to eat again, you won't go ballistic.

2. Portion off the plate into thirds.

This is a tried and true method of controlling how much you eat. You must measure the proportions of what you are ingesting. You really need to focus on three types of food groups when you eat:

- Carbohydrates

- Proteins

- Vegetables

Follow these suggested plate percentage divisions in order to manage your calories better.

MEAL	CARBOHYDRATES	PROTEINS	VEGETABLES
Breakfast	50 percent, largest percentage of the day	30 percent	20 percent, least percentage of the day
Lunch	30 percent	20 percent, least percentage of the day	50 percent, largest percentage of the day

MEAL	CARBOHYDRATES	PROTEINS	VEGETABLES
Dinner	10–15 percent, least percentage of the day	55–60 percent	30 percent

You need fewer carbohydrates at night so that your body can have less available energy to begin repairing itself from the long day and after exercise. It has to repair those torn muscle fibers and start building new ones. Make it *look* for stored energy in fat cells. Don't load your stomach with carbohydrates or you defeat the purpose. Instead, load the carbohydrates early in the day because you need to ramp up your metabolism, and then begin to taper off throughout the day, increasing the things that you will need the most: protein and vegetables. The protein will be broken down and utilized to build the muscle while the vegetables are the secret ingredient to sending your metabolism into overdrive.

Vegetables help to:

- Provide the body with calcium (strong bones) and other vitamins such as A, B, C, and K

- Increase antioxidant levels—necessary elements that help protect the human body from oxidant stress, diseases, and cancers, and develop the capacity to fight against these by boosting immunity

- Move fecal matter from the body. Vegetables are packed with soluble as well as insoluble dietary fiber known as nonstarch polysaccharides (NSP) such as cellulose, mucilage, hemi-cellulose, gums, and pectin. These substances absorb excess water in the colon and retain a good amount of moisture in the fecal matter, making it easier to pass from the body, which protects you from conditions like hemorrhoids, colon cancer, chronic constipation, and rectal fissures.

3. Eat six times a day, but space it out every three hours.

Now before you go telling everyone that I released you to go on an eating spree, read a little more here. You must eat more times a day so that your stomach works out during the day. The more your stomach has to work to digest what you are eating, the more calories it burns, the more energy is expended over time, and the more your substances are broken down and expelled from the body naturally.

With this, your new way of eating is now contributing to your successfully increasing your metabolism. This is the one time that double-dipping is acceptable. Eat more, burn more. Just make sure you eat the big three meals and add snacks in between breakfast, lunch, and at the end of dinner.

What snacks? you ask. They mainly come from the list I am providing of the ten foods that help to increase metabolism and enhance your body's ability to be healthy. You can also add a protein shake, protein bar, or Greek yogurt (must have at least double-digit grams of protein in it) to the list. If you were to overindulge in one thing, I'd rather have it be protein because the body will get rid of it when it is an overabundance.

4. Count your calories.

There has always been a huge debate as to how many calories you need to consume daily, because the body has energy needs that must be fulfilled. These come in the form of calories. Three systems of the body are battling for calories:

digestion, daily living (heart, lung, and skin repair), and the energy needed to work out.

A gentleman by the name of Alan Aragon came up with an equation that is both simple to follow and easy to apply. He has more than twenty years of success in the fitness field and earned his bachelor and master of science in nutrition with top honors. Alan provides continuing education for the Commission on Dietetic Registration, National Academy of Sports Medicine, and National Strength and Conditioning Association. He designs programs for recreational, olympic, and professional athletes, including the Los Angeles Lakers, Los Angeles Kings, and Anaheim Mighty Ducks. He is the nutrition advisor of *Men's Health* magazine.[2]

Alan recommends taking your body weight and multiplying it by 10. That's the number of calories your body needs daily, just to operate. Now if you exercise during the week, take the number of days per week that you work out and add it to 10, then multiply your weight by that number. Then, subtract 500 from it. For example: if you weigh 150 pounds and work out three times a week, multiply 150 by 13, and then subtract 500. You should consume roughly 1,450 calories daily.[3] That is, if you are trying to lose weight. If you want to maintain, keep the 500. The majority of the calories that you will lose out on will be from digestion because the other systems are in dire need of them. That way, your body can maintain its normal functions while providing the appropriate amount of calories it needs to optimize the workout energy expenditures.

Ten Foods to Jump Start Your Metabolism

Drumroll, please. Here is a list of the ten foods that are going to jump start that meandering metabolism, fortify your body with nutrients to maximize your healing, and turn you into a mean, lean, healthy machine. Your body will transition from a slow-going, tip-toeing slug to a confident, show-stopping, and strutting stud in no time.

1. Cinnamon

Cinnamon helps blood sugar get into cells to be used for energy, so less is stored as fat. One-fourth to one teaspoon added to something you eat daily will do.

2. Green tea

Green tea has caffeine, which raises your heart rate, compelling your system to burn calories faster. It also has catechins, substances that assist in burning belly fat. Aim for three eight-ounce cups a day.

3. Chili peppers

Found in hot salsa, and Thai, Indian, and Chinese curry dishes, chili peppers are packed with capsaicin, which increases your body temperature somewhat, giving your metabolism an extra calorie-burning push. Two teaspoons is generally considered a safe serving size, but it all depends on your tolerance. If you cook chili peppers into a dish, you may need more to increase the fiery flavor. One serving of chili peppers should suffice.

4. Chicken and fish

Remember that I said it takes energy to digest food? Well, your body burns more calories digesting and metabolizing protein than it does while breaking down carbohydrates and fats, so this may help keep your metabolism revving away long after you finish eating your meal.

5. Yogurt (Greek, please)

Yogurt contains probiotics—that's the *friendly* bacteria that helps to clean out your digestive system. The key to losing weight is to minimize the number of calories you consume. Naturally, nonfat plain yogurt is a better alternative than low-fat because it has fewer calories due to the absence of fat. Stay away from flavored yogurts because they contain more sugar, and thus more calories. Greek is king—it has about the same number of calories as regular yogurt but contains more calcium.

6. Grapes

Rich in vitamins A, B_6, C, and B_9 (or folate) grapes activate your metabolism, help prevent heart disease, breast cancer, kidney disorders, Alzheimer's disease, and other illnesses. A handful of grapes will do.

7. Pears

A great source of soluble dietary fiber, pears are rich in vitamins E, C, B_2, copper, and potassium (battles against cramping muscles). They are also a good source of antioxidants and can help relieve inflammation, throat problems, and fever. One pear will do the trick.

These next three are what I term "fitness builders." We can also refer to them as illness buffers. They are good sources of building and sustaining an optimal level of health and fitness.

8. Pomegranates

Eating pomegranate seeds for at least three months seems to halt the hardening of the arteries (atherosclerosis). Type 2 diabetics have more problems with the development of this disease than those without type 2 diabetes. The juice from the seeds appears to halt atherosclerosis by lowering high blood cholesterol levels. Research also shows that eating organic pomegranate seeds and drinking pomegranate juice can increase oxygen levels to the heart, which is great for heart attack survivors, those suffering from atherosclerosis and COPD.

They are a good source of vitamin B_6 and vitamin C. Vitamin C is well known for its healthy promotion of blood vessel strength. Low vitamin B_6 levels have been linked to higher homocysteine levels in heart attack and stroke victims.

Pomegranates are also known to:

- Combat the build-up of dental plaque

- Naturally suppress diarrhea

- Ease and/or eliminate different symptoms of menopause

- Work to buffer the effects of free radical damage to your cells caused by oxidation (volatile processes between atoms), which produces free radicals. These by-products of functions that occur within the body and various elements outside of the body, such as radiation from the sun, can cause serious damage. These powerful little seeds help to neutralize the effects of free radicals.

9. Celery

An excellent source of vitamin C (protection against immune system deficiencies, cardiovascular disease, prenatal health problems, and eye disease) and fiber (metabolism booster), celery is also a very good source of potassium, folic acid, and vitamins B_6 and B_1 (antioxidants to fight against cancer-causing free radicals). Celery is filled with vitamin B_2 (a metabolism booster that keeps nerves and blood cells healthy).

The properties in celery also provide healing for:

- Bladder infections—With loads of analgesic, anti-inflammatory and diuretic compounds, as well as some calcium blockers, celery seeds are said to improve the quantity and quality of urine and are a useful diuretic for urinary tract infections (UTIs).

- Bursitis—COX-2 inhibitors are a type of non-steroidal anti-inflammatory drugs (NSAIDs) that were acclaimed as the new *miracle aspirin*. Celery is one of the best known sources of these COX-2 inhibitors. So bursitis and other inflammatory conditions benefit from celery. Try making a tea from freshly crushed celery seeds, or take celery seed supplements.

- Gout—The COX-2 inhibitors present in celery and celery seeds are also good at reducing uric acid levels, which are the cause of gout attacks. Try the tea method again by pouring boiling water over one teaspoon of freshly crushed celery seeds and letting it steep for ten to twenty minutes before drinking it. Juicing is not a bad option as freshly squeezed celery juice on its own provides just enough assistance.

• Cancer—Phytochemical coumarin is a compound that has been proven effective in cancer prevention. It also enhances the activity of certain white blood cells that help fight cancer, preventing those pesky free radicals from damaging cells. Another compound, acetylene, has been shown to stop the growth of tumor cells. Phenolic acids block the action of hormone-like substances called prostaglandins, which have been known to encourage the growth of tumor cells. All of these healing substances are found in celery.

• Fungal infections—Celery acts as a natural resistant to pathogens during storage because it contains a melting pot of fungicides, with more than two dozen already identified. Research suggests eating one celery stalk a day to keep those microbes in check.

• Allergies—Celery is wealthy in certain acids, sterols, and flavonoids that assist in providing anti-inflammatory responses. Thus, it indirectly helps to reduce the body's response to allergens.

• High blood pressure—Phytochemical compounds present in celery called coumarins are able to tone the vascular system, which lowers blood pressure.

• Indigestion—Celery contains two dozen painkillers, more than two dozen anti-inflammatories, eleven anti-ulcer compounds, and more than two dozen sedatives to complement the activities of its three carminative compounds. These are herbs or preparations that prevent or facilitate expulsion of gas.

* Memory loss—Celery contains a compound called luteolin, which is showing promise for lowering levels of plaque-forming proteins in the brain.

10. Peanuts

Peanuts are packed with fiber and protein. Fiber forces your stomach to stay active during the day and night in the digestive process. The more your body/stomach work, the more energy is consumed. This helps to shed off unnecessary calories that would otherwise be stored as fat. The protein is needed to help your body rebuild and repair muscle that is torn and damaged during a good workout. They also keep you satisfied and full for a long time (fiber). This helps you to manage your hunger. Some suggest that the urge to eat is stifled for as much as two-and-a-half hours versus the half hour you'll get from high-carbohydrate foods.

> Resting energy expenditures of peanut and peanut butter eaters normally run higher than those who don't consume them.

Peanuts can also (like the other nine foods listed) increase your metabolic rate. Resting energy expenditures of peanut and peanut butter eaters normally run higher than those who don't consume them—these can be as much as double-digit percent increases after regular peanut consumption compared with those who don't.

The fat in peanuts is the good stuff (HDLs). They help

provide satiety and add a little to the taste buds so you don't feel deprived.

Managing your blood sugar when trying to eat right is huge! Peanuts are known to help stabilize your blood sugar with their low glycemic index. They are digested more slowly, releasing sugar gradually into the bloodstream. This helps you to avoid going nuts and mistakenly eating a piece of cake or a handful of cookies to satisfy your craving for sugar.

Also, I love the way they provide long-lasting energy bursts. You can pound out more workouts in the gym and tone up for that summer body.

Following these dietary recommendations of controlling your plate size, managing your portions, consuming the seven super foods and three fitness builders, eating five to six times a day, and calorie counting will swing the pendulum back in your favor in the battle against the bulge. You can do it. It's just going to take a little more focus.

Chapter 6

IF YOU'RE NOT GIVING, THEN YOU'RE NOT GETTING

I N THE LAST section I talked about the importance of getting your spiritual balance. For many people, the battle of the bulge is a battle that first and foremost takes place in the mind. Once you have overcome the stinking thinking that drives you to the refrigerator for that big bowl of ice cream, or to the pantry for the supersized bag of potato chips, you will discover that the fruit of the Spirit not only brings the possibility of wholeness and health to you, but they put within your heart a desire to reach out to others. You change from being a person who is only interested in getting—"It's all about ME!"— to being a person who cares more about giving to others.

Putting that desire to help others to work right now, while you are still in the process of overcoming your own overweight and poor health patterns, will give you even more motivation to stay with the plan until you have reached your goal of wholeness and health. So let's look closer at this new powerful motivator of *giving*.

The Power of a Mind That Wants to Give

Giving without regard of ever getting back—what a virtuous way of thinking. You really have to be plugged in to something bigger than yourself to believe in such a way. Don't we all wish to strive to such selfless perfection? I believe that deep within us, underneath all the layers of hurt, insecurity, self-indulgence, and self-preservation, there lies an innate ability to care for others more than ourselves.

> The battle of the bulge is a battle that first and foremost takes place in the mind.

But something happened along the way that makes us pull back the helpful hand to our brother, sister, neighbor, and friend in order to preserve the one thing that matters most: ourselves. Have you ever watched children play together? It's incredible how early on in life this principle rears its ugly head. Picture it: sand box, three to four children are involved in corporate play time, each one possessing their favorite toy. One child (child one) decides that his or her toy is no longer of any value and begins to covet another child's toy (child two). Child one slowly meanders forward, creeping closer and closer to the desired object. Child two finds something else that momentarily occupies his attention and turns away. That's when it happens—child one takes the toy and retreats back to his or her respective play space, hopeful that child two will not take notice.

But child two does, and then follows child one with the sole intent of retrieving his lost item. Of course the words, "Mine, mine, *mine!*" spill out of the mouth of each child as they wrestle to obtain the prize, each one screaming at the top of his or her lungs as if it's the last toy left on the playground.

But something else interesting happens. Child two notices a new toy; the toy that child one discarded. Child two picks it up and starts to play with it. Guess you can figure out what happens next. Child one drops the newly gained toy and immediately goes for the toy that child two has that used to be his. Child one only finds it to be of value now because someone else does. Child one could decide to share the toy until child two grows tired of it, but it would be at the risk of missing out on something that may be of greater gain in the not too distant future. Or, maybe child one feels as though he may be taken advantage of by child two in the future if he interprets kindness as weakness, and so decides to continually take toys from child two.

It is natural to elicit this sort of behavior because it derives from primitive survival skills. If I do something for someone and do not get anything back, it makes me look weak. Have you been there before?

Are you the child on the playground, making rounds to obtain all that you desire, without a second thought of giving first? The thing that gets us in trouble with this way of thinking is our motives. We are looking for something in return, rather than giving with a pure heart.

I'd like to pay homage to a woman who gave diligently without regard of gaining anything in return. Florence Nightingale (yes, I went there) was a celebrated English nurse, writer, and statistician. She pioneered her works of giving during her time as a nurse in the Crimean War, while she tended to wounded soldiers. Although she was born into a rich, upper-class, well-connected British family at the Villa

Colombia, she understood the value of not thinking of herself higher than anyone else. She focused more on the act of service. Against her family's best wishes, Florence entered into nursing in 1844. She later said that she was inspired by a calling from God saying: "God called me in the morning and asked me would I do good for him alone without reputation."[1]

Despite the anger and distress of her mother and sister, she rebelled against the expected role for a woman of her status to become a wife and mother. Against the opposition of her family and the chauvinistic societal expectations of women (especially affluent English ones), she followed her calling and set out to change the world. Her team of thirty-eight female nurses arrived in Crimea and set up camp, reporting back to Britain about the horrific conditions for the wounded. She asserted that the poor care for wounded soldiers was being delivered by overworked medical staff. Medicines were in short supply, hygiene was neglected, and the high prevalence of infection was commonplace.

> "God called me in the morning and asked me would I do good for him alone without reputation."
> —FLORENCE NIGHTINGALE

Florence sent a plea to *The Times* (a prominent newspaper company in Britain) for a government solution to the poor condition of the facilities. The British government designed a prefabricated hospital, built in England and shipped to the Dardanelles. The result was Renkioi Hospital, a civilian facility that had a death rate less than one-tenth that of Scutari.[2] Those soldiers could not provide anything to Florence in return for her exemplary behavior.

Florence gained a nickname for her contribution during the Crimean War: "The Lady With the Lamp." It was reported that: "She is a 'ministering angel' without any exaggeration in these hospitals...every poor fellow's face softens with gratitude at the sight of her. When all the medical officers have retired for the night...she may be observed alone, with a little lamp in her hand, making her solitary rounds."[3]

Her dedication to a calling of selflessness and moral duty gave a sense of greater accomplishment. She could have easily settled to live out her days of affluent living without impacting anyone else, but she chose a different path. And for that, she lived a healthy life, all the way until the age of ninety, without regard for reputation.

Giving without the expectation of getting anything back helps everyone. Your mind and soul will be rewarded with the gratitude and satisfaction of inspiring someone else to think outside of themselves. Hopefully, they too will do the same for someone else.

COSBY'S CORNER
Why You Shouldn't Trust Yourself

OK, let's take a quick break from reflecting on how selfish you are. I don't want to torment you or overstate my point on that topic. Besides, you have so much more to focus on right now. You're trying to get yourself right as it pertains to the mind, body, and spirit, right? So let's switch gears to talking about how greedy you are. Yeah, I said it: selfish and greedy. I see the connection, even if you do not. Just kidding. Don't put the book down, please. No, really, I mean it. You started on this journey, and you are going to finish it. Even if you feel beaten down by the time you complete reading it.

I want this section of Cosby's Corner to be an opportunity for me to issue a challenge to you. This is going to be a line in the sand moment. It centers around one of my pet peeves—buffets. I can't stand buffets. They are the kiss of death to a person trying to make life changes concerning eating. You must understand one thing and one thing alone about buffets: you are setting yourself up for failure if you go. The phrase "all you can eat" makes my stomach turn because I know the emotion it evokes in certain individuals.

Before you go getting all mad at me, I must make a confession first. I used to love them. Yes, that's right. My name is Braxton A. Cosby, and I too was a buffet addict. Man, there wasn't anything better than going to a buffet. Think about it for a second. It has everything you want—unlimited food, drinks, and desert. To top it all off, someone actually cleans up after you so that you do not have to waste any extra energy by taking your tray and discarding it. You can put all of your efforts into eating some more. You can just sit back, eat, relax, and of course, eat again, again, and again.

I found out quickly that feeling like my belly button was about to pop off and slap the person across the table from me was not the way to go, nor was it cool.

If you are laughing or getting totally grossed out by now (I hope you are doing both), then hopefully I am making my point. You may be on your way to a breakthrough moment. There is no way to successfully go to a buffet and calorie count your way to safety. Come on, man! Don't fool yourself. It is not going to happen! Do not trust yourself. Step away from the buffet table and find sanctuary at the salad bar of some other restaurant.

You can't take a kleptomaniac to the Tower of London, leave him alone in the room with the Crown Jewels, and not expect him to attempt a five-finger discount.

He is going to leave with a little something-something in his pockets.

I expect the same for you. "I just wanted a little sample. A little bite won't hurt," you say. Right. Keep believing that you have the willpower to stop after one bite. Before you know it, you will be cradled in the corner, feet sprawled out in front of you, stomach stuffed to the brink of exploding, with your psyche shattered because you lost the battle once more.

The best way not to get burned is not to dance around the fire. Don't take unnecessary chances with this, people. Repeat after me: "I am a person with no self-control. If I weren't, I would not be reading this book in the first place." Amen. Now, doesn't that feel better? Leave the buffets to the folks in denial. Don't hate me. I'm just issuing a challenge, and I'm just saying . . .

■■■

Teach Your Spirit to Give Out of the Resources God Has Given You

Back to the serious stuff now, the spiritual side of things. As referenced earlier in the section about Florence Nightingale, giving is always the best thing to do, period. When you give, without expectation, something happens inside of you. It stabs at the inner selfish desire to obtain and hoard, and releases the ability to look at the condition of the other person. This way of thinking is critical to provide the foundation of God to provide for you. When you give without expecting anything else in return, you are telling God that you trust Him to provide for you.

> When you give, without expectation, it stabs at the inner selfish desire to obtain and hoard.

This is a concept you need to put into practice right now, right in the middle of your journey from overweight to healthy. God has given you the resources through the fruit of the Spirit to be successful with your own spiritual journey. Now He is asking you to move away from your former mind-set of, "Me first, me most, me always," to a new personal identity of *Giver.*

You are asking the Holy Spirit to replenish your resources so that you don't have to be distracted with the task of figuring out how to get it back. You can then focus on staying kingdom minded and follow the example set by that of no other than Jesus Christ Himself. He allowed Himself to be a sacrifice for a lineage of people that He would never see, or may never personally know, just because He loved you. This was done because He sees you as being bigger than yourself through the eyes of a just and caring God. Although God wants us to follow His example, this was also a commandment: love your neighbor as yourself. This mind-set was first decreed, and then Jesus Himself gave provision for the propagating system of man taking care of one another. He no longer has to intercede on our behalf.

We see this in Luke 6:38:

> Give, and it will be given to you: Good measure, pressed down, shaken together, and running over will men give unto you. For with the measure you use, it will be measured unto you.

Sit back and think about this verse for a moment before you read any further. God has set a system in place that runs itself while He takes care of the rest of the universe. If people give to one another (you give to others), a good measure that is shaken together (combined with things that you didn't even imagine being given back to you), and running over (more than you gave initially) will be poured into your lap. This is huge. God didn't say that He would give to us because we gave to someone else. He says that others will give back to you on a level that supersedes the original act of giving.

Therefore you can undeniably know for sure that when you give to someone, your Father in heaven will see it and send the exact measure of spiritual inspiration and consideration to someone else to act in obedience and bless you above measure. You will see the fruit of your sowing in the here and now. What a great reward for your service. Not only will you see others get blessed, lives changed, and circumstances improved, but you will receive the overflowing increase of a provisional system that was spoken into existence by the Son of God Himself. Now that's powerful: want more for others than what you want for yourself. Stop being so selfish, and start giving back. If you want to have success in all areas of your life, you must first want those things for others, and then God can pour into you from the abundance that He has.

Body Truth: It's All About Physics

I made this one as basic as possible. The scientific research behind the principle of giving is credited to Sir Isaac Newton. Formally stated, it's Newton's Third Law: For every action, there is an equal and opposite reaction. How about that? With all that Newton was coming up with way back then, never did he know that there would be some application to how we as a society should interact with one another. He just thought he was dealing with some simple physics (oxymoron—no such thing as simple physics). But think about all the things that we discussed in this chapter:

- Florence Nightingale's selfless actions to obey a calling and save the lives of thousands of soldiers

- You letting someone else cut in front of you in the buffet line as you put down your plate and step away

- Christ's example of how we should act toward one another

It all adds up. We are not just beings who are here for the sole purpose of standing by and watching as the world, solar system, galaxy, and universe carry on in their evolutionary pathways. We are meant to be active participants in the journey. We are commanded by a higher being, a chief Creator, to assist in its expansion.

The growth of every individual on Earth is not fixed; it is dynamic, and it is dependent upon the events of the people who exist within the moments. You have the power to act, the free will to serve, and the liberty to answer a calling (just like Florence did) to the symbolic cogwheel in the circuit that affects the outcome of the world itself. There would not be heroes in a world where everyone stands up and does what they are supposed to do. It would be an equal playing field, in which one hand washes another, one person lifts the other up, and families and nations encourage one another to make the better decisions of putting aside their wants for the needs of others.

For every action, there is an equal and opposite reaction. This means that for every good and bad measure, there is an equal opposite bad and good measure. For every negative and positive, there is positive and negative. We have the key to the equation. Life is not the summation of just physics and time, but it is the culmination of an individual's free will choices and the motive that follows behind those choices.

So right now, right in the middle of your journey to overcome the self-motivation that caused you to need to deal with the issue of weight loss, begin the lifelong identity of being a giver. While you are using the resources God is giving to you to be victorious on your personal journey, reach out of yourself to give those resources to someone else who desperately needs your gift.

> You have the power to act, the free will to serve, and the liberty to answer a calling to the symbolic cogwheel in the circuit that affects the outcome of the world itself.

I am issuing a challenge to you again. Give freely, out of the love that I know exists within you. Act as if the world—no, the universe—depended on your solitary performance. Know that you can live with the assurance that you have played your part in the provisional laws that govern the universe. You have the power to do more, be more, and influence more in the lives of people than you've ever known. What are you going to do about it?

Chapter 7

EMBRACE YOUR POWER

Y OU HAVE THE power! Repeat that to yourself three times before you read any further. Now that you've had the chance to let it settle in, you have the opportunity to come to the place of understanding—the understanding that no matter how challenging situations may appear, or how impossible the task before you may seem to be, you have the power to get through it. I'm not promising that you will always excel at it, but embrace the idea that you have the potential inside of you to see the light at the end of the tunnel, stay the course, and make it to the other side.

Life can throw the kitchen sink at you, along with the plumbing, the blueprint, and the water bill, and you if you hold on to the faintest of all hope, things will work out in your favor.

Use the Power of a Sound Mind

When it comes to life's trials, most people give up and walk away right before the moment of their breakthrough. They were right on the cusp of receiving the good news, but they lost the one thing we have all been given freely to wield like a sharp sword: *hope*. I know this to be true, and after reading this short testimony, hopefully you will believe as well.

> Speaking of diet, he and six other men had to share a loaf of bread, with each man rotating the cutting duties daily to assure that everyone got an even take.

During the course of my career in geriatrics, I came across a delightful man who shared a story with me about true hope and conviction. This fellow was an old army war veteran now in his late eighties. He served in World War II, and in 1944 he and his platoon were captured by the Germans. More than two hundred soldiers were ambushed and overcome by a small battalion of German troops in the Battle of the Bulge on Christmas Eve.

Prior to being captured, an explosion erupted nearby, sending shrapnel into his head and arm. He survived his minor wounds and lived the next four and a half months in a prison camp, where he lived off of nothing but a two-meal-a-day regimen of bread and soup.

He slept in a barrack of three-level bunks that supported six men. He was forced to sleep back to back with another fellow soldier on a wooden bed with no mattress and only one sheet. Speaking of diet, he and six other men had to share a loaf of bread, with each man rotating the cutting duties daily to assure that everyone got an even take. He had just been recently married prior to being deployed overseas, and to make matters worse, he was only able to write two letters to his new bride; only one of which was actually delivered to her.

Over that span of the four and a half months, he lost a little over fifty pounds. A small laceration on his hand developed an infection that burned with searing heat. He only received two showers during his capture and was made to stand outside for up to two hours a day in the January and February German winter while the barracks was swept clean.

He finally got a taste of freedom when the news broke that the Russians were pressing from the east and the Allied forces were marching in from the west. The German leaders ordered the German officers to take the troop into a concealed corridor in the forest where they spent the next thirty days camping in abandoned barn houses.

> I never lost the conviction that I would make it back home.

With the fear of being bombed by Allied troops scratching at the back of his mind, he held out hope that it would all be over soon. When he finally received his true freedom and the German regime had fallen, he headed back home to his spouse.

Can you imagine being captured; imprisoned with no food, no fresh clothes, and no bath; and separated from the love of your life without any clue that the war would be over, much less anyone come to rescue you for over four months? I asked him the one question that fed on my own level of sanity: "How did you make it through?"

He simply answered, "I never lost the conviction that I would make it back home."

Wow! He maintained conviction in the face of true calamity. I was amazed. His testimony illustrated the power of maintaining the conviction that there is purpose for our struggles and somehow injecting the hope that our negative circumstances will one day get better. It was an inspiration for me in my personal life struggles. I used it to motivate me to accomplish the few meager tasks I had set before me—one being to finish writing this book and pursuing this calling from God to write.

> Life's victories are rarely easy, but if you are able to somehow ride the rugged waves, you can land on peaceable shores that hold prosperity and happier moments.

What is it that you are wrestling with in your daily life? Is it something that weighs heavily on you, making life seem abysmal? Think of the story of the unnamed soldier. Putting his story into perspective may give you the push you need to stand up under the pressure and overcome. Life's victories are rarely easy, but if you are able to somehow ride the rugged waves, you can land on peaceable shores that hold prosperity and happier moments.

COSBY'S CORNER
The Dog That Walked on Water

There once was a guy who was always negative about everything. His vantage point of life rested somewhere between the floor and the dust covering it. He believed that there was always a dark lining to every cloud. If you looked up the word pessimist in the dictionary, you'd find his name (but not his photograph, because he would have removed it, proclaiming that it was the worst picture ever). He brought down everybody around him. He once said that if you received money in your tax return, it was just a setup from the government to come after you the following year.

One day, a different man went duck hunting. He had recently purchased a brand-new, duck-retrieving hunting dog; the owner promised him that he was in for a real treat. He shot down his first duck and whistled for the dog to retrieve the duck from the water. To his surprise, the dog not only retrieved the duck faster than any other dog before it, it walked on top of the water rather than swim.

The man was amazed. He quickly loaded his gun and shot down three more ducks. To his surprise, the dog did it again, skating on top of the water with ease and scooping up the three ducks with razor sharp precision every time. He was so thrilled that he decided he would take the negative man with him on the next duck hunting trip.

The next month, he invited the negative man hunting with him. They loaded their rifles and began to shoot. Like clockwork, three ducks came crashing from the sky, and the dog sprang from the boat, jogged on top of the water, and returned to the boat with three ducks in tow. The hunter looked at the negative man awaiting his response. The negative man's jaw dropped in amazement. The hunter asked him, "So what do you think about that?"

The negative man took a long hard swallow, clearing his throat before speaking. "Well, I must admit. I am truly taken back. I can't believe what I just saw."

The hunter was thrilled. Finally there was something that the negative man couldn't have a negative comment about. He found something to confound his negativism. It was a breakthrough. "Right, isn't it incredible?" he asked.

"Yeah, I never thought I'd see the day that a duck-retrieval dog couldn't swim."

I hope you got that joke. But seriously, aren't there people out in the world just like that, driven to see only the negative aspects of life, never considering the positive side? I give them credit for being totally sold out in their belief. While I hope you aren't one of these people, what if we could tap into that degree of conviction? We'd be moving mountains, feeding the homeless, and saving the world, way too busy to worry about being overweight. Let's try to cross over into the deep waters of faith. Who knows, you may find your inner duck-retrieving dog and walk on water. I'm just saying . . .

■■■

The Power of the Spirit Within You

I've talked a lot about the word *power* and the influence it has on all of our lives. That is because I believe it to be something that is real. It's tangible. It does not just exist in a realm that is untouchable, like some ghost or cloud in the sky. This *power* can be manipulated and held in the palm of your hand, to be wielded like a sword. It can cut and destroy things like evil principalities that attempt to reign over your life and devour you, trying to convince you that you have no purpose, that you are somehow just an irrelevant person who is meant to stand on the sideline and let the rest of the world do marvelous works.

> You are more than just a spectator. God has given you the divine appointment to be a difference maker.

You are more than just a spectator. God has given you the divine appointment to be a difference maker. You have a spiritual gift resting inside of you, lying dormant, and beckoning to be called out of its slumber. This spiritual power is meant to be made manifest to bless other people while being a blessing to you, all the while exalting and magnifying the glory of God.

But you and I both know that I can talk about this until I am blue in the face, and it wouldn't mean a hill of beans if you do not come alongside me and walk in the same conviction that my words are true, that they have meaning. This *calling* on your life that I speak about is not mere myth and fantasy but a real token of the reflection of the plan of God. What God has set in place for the

> Losing weight, being released from terminal illness, and recovering from diseases are nothing more than bricks and concrete that build our individual platforms of faith so that others can be encouraged by us.

world is happening, with or without the aid of a single person. But what an amazing opportunity has been shared with us in partnering with God for the pursuit of His children. We are invited to participate in working out the plan of salvation.

You have to rise up first. Determine in your mind (soul) that the Spirit that dwells within you is the source of the power and that you really want to use it for God's purpose. In fulfilling that purpose we are able to perform miracles, signs, and wonders. These three things are not only for the world, but for us.

Losing weight, being released from terminal illness and recovering from diseases are nothing more than bricks and concrete that build our individual platforms of faith so that others can be encouraged by us. In 2 Timothy 1:7 Paul declares, "For God has not given us the spirit of fear, but of power, and love, and self-control." That same spirit that Paul is referring to is composed of three things: power, love, and self-discipline. This forms the nucleus of the substance necessary for accepting your purpose and releasing your faith. You need these three things to accomplish your goals.

You can no longer be comfortable wearing the wardrobe of dreariness and despair, doom and gloom. You need a fresh change, a new perspective. One that is based on truth and the following:

- *Power* to overcome your old self, along with the bad habits you developed that have trapped you and created the person you are today.

- *Love* to accept the things about you that are not changeable and to fortify the things that can be improved upon, creating an atmosphere of hope. Loving yourself, God, and the people around you allows for His will to be perfected in us.

- *Self-discipline* to say no to the things that hurt you and yes to turning the page in a new chapter of your life that is filled with peace and joy.

The truth is that if you change the patterning of your negative thinking (*stinking thinking*) and begin to think on only the victory, God will not only help you, but He will also hand the victory to you. In Paul's letter to the Philippians he advises us to change our thinking when he says:

Finally, brothers, whatever things are true, whatever things are honest, whatever things are just, whatever things are pure, whatever things are lovely, whatever things are of good report, if there is any virtue, and if there is any praise, think on these things.

—PHILIPPIANS 4:8

Paul knew that no one is able to get anywhere in this world with his or her mind clouded by inimical thoughts. He urges us to think on things that reflect truth, nobility, righteousness, purity, love, admiration, excellence, and praise. With these you will be fully equipped to thwart the plans of the wicked one *and win*—win in your homes, win at work, win in your relationships, and, most of all, win the battle within yourself.

> Add God in every exercise, every repetition/set, food choice, and negative habit in order to propel yourself beyond your own limiting expectations.

Once you manage to bring yourself into God's truth concerning positive thinking, you then are able to bring your labors into fruition. In everything you do, acknowledge that your strength comes from Christ and your belief in Him. There are no longer barriers, defeats, losses, or failures, only successes and accomplishments for those who believe. You need only to add God in every exercise, every repetition/set, food choice, and negative habit in order to propel yourself beyond your own limiting expectations.

The Power Link of Body and Mind

I know, I know. Maybe you're not totally convinced about the link between sound thinking and healing. Well, science has proven time and time again that the ability to *feel* better comes from the commitment to *think* better. In no other platform do we see this phenomenon more than in sports.

Those athletes who seem to be *in the zone* are actively tapping into that power. They only appear to be unstoppable because they believe that they are. This even goes beyond the playing field and into the infirmary. In a study conducted at Florida State University, researcher Lydia Ievleva of the Department of Physical Education, and Terry Orlick of the University of Ottawa, conducted a survey to determine whether athletes who healed very rapidly demonstrated greater evidence than did slower healing athletes of psychosocial factors thought to be related to healing.

A sample was taken of thirty-nine prescreened individuals who met injury criteria of ligament sprains in either the knee or ankle. Subjects were asked to complete a survey that measured certain factors such as positive attitude, outlook, stress and stress control, social support, goal setting, positive self-talk, and mental imagery. Other items scored reflected belief and recommendations for enhanced healing.

> Thinking positively fosters positive changes, whether it is related to healing or performance outcomes.

The twenty-five question survey asked direct questions about the injury and recovery with a range score of 0-10. Along with the survey, a physiotherapist's assessment was provided to rank the athlete's recovery (three groups: fast healers, average healers, and slow healers). Overall, those athletes that provided more positive answers to active variables such as positive self-talk, goal setting, and healing imagery were the most closely associated with the fast-healing group.[1]

In April of 2011, another systematic search of PubMed

was conducted by a group of researchers to find articles that reflected the effect of psychological variables on early surgical recovery. Out of sixteen articles found, fifteen reported a significant association between at least one psychological variable or intervention and early postoperative outcomes.[2] In fact, the article cites that dispositional optimism, religiousness, anger control, low pain expectations, and external locus of control seemed to promote healing.

The evidence supports the assumptions. Thinking positively fosters positive changes, whether it is related to healing or performance outcomes. There's no guarantee that the journey is going to be easy, but you can rest assured that retraining yourself to be more in conjunction with attitudes and beliefs that mirror desirable results can only make it that much more rewarding.

Chapter 8

CONNECT WITH YOUR PURPOSE

H OW DO YOU find your purpose? It's a loaded question, for sure. Some may go through their entire lives living for themselves, day to day, same job, same group of friends, making money, attaining things, and achieving goals, but never realizing what any of it means. They may have accomplished something arbitrarily by happenstance—right place, right person, and right time. There was never a plan or structure to what they did, yet they were able to create opportunity out of nothing. Plenty of people have done it before. That's all well and good, but if you are going to be the best person you want to be, you have to have a plan. Find a purpose.

Losing weight just because someone else thinks you should or because your STATS don't line up is all well and good. You may actually meet your goals early on, but the staying power will come from finding purpose for what you are doing. Success in nearly anything is only sus-

> If you are going to be the best person you want to be, you have to have a plan.

tained if the people behind it truly believe in what they do and have passion for it. That passion is founded on the principles of purpose.

So I ask you again: How do you find your purpose?

Use Your Mind to Define Your Purpose

I think it has to start with defining what the word *purpose* means to you. Purpose is the end to the means. Keeping with the theme of this book, let's think about it on the terms of eating. You eat for many reasons, but ultimately it is to fulfill something that you desire. At the root of it all, eating is essential to take in nutrients that the body needs to heal itself, for growth, diges-

> Success in nearly anything is only sustained if the people behind it truly believe in what they do and have passion for it.

tion, and to fuel the energy systems of the body, which make it all possible. Let's face it, without food you would ultimately die. So eating has purpose—real purpose, with negative consequences if you were to go without. Now let's look at life and its purpose, the purpose that you are now going to define for yourself.

If you have not yet found your purpose, fear not because I'm sure that you are not alone. Many people of all age groups are floating through life just making do. As a matter of fact, I recently began to piece together the parts of my life that construct the purpose that God has for me to fulfill. God wants to use all of us for something. But do not get this confused: God does not *need* any of us to do anything that He wants to be done. He can do it all by Himself.

But He does desire to have us work in accordance with His plans so that He can be glorified through our successes, failures, and testimonies. Sometimes the purpose that we are trying to create seems brilliant. We identify an opportunity that seems picture perfect for God to deliver on. It might be some last-minute phone call to the bank to stop your foreclosure, or a relieving answer from the doctor concerning your recent tests results. Or maybe it's an encouraging word that you need to hear from your spouse or children about how amazing you are. But alas, how many of us know that the best made plans of mice and men really don't make the grade when it comes to God's all-knowing, all-consuming purpose in our lives? He loves to make new things out of new circumstances using His children.

The Bible is full of amazing testimonies about David, Samson, Daniel, Ruth, Abraham, and the disciples. Why in the world God used Peter, of all people, to preach on the Day of Pentecost is beyond me. But it was marvelous, and at the end of it all, only God could get the glory. That's why He does it the way He does. God's fresh anointing is best manifested in newness, not in carbon copies or facsimiles that allow man to claim the victory.

Discovering God's Purpose for My Life

I'd like to share with you the purpose that God gave me. At the age of nineteen, I was ranked in the top for both the 10 and 400 meter hurdles. It was my dream to be an elite athlete in either football or track and field. Slowly but surely, I was living out at least one of them. I was a late bloomer, only starting to compete in organized sports in the tenth grade, but I had made great strides. My God-given talent had carried me a long way, and in 1996 I earned a silver medal in the Junior Pan American Games in the 400 meter hurdles. I later transferred from the University of Miami to Louisiana State University on a full scholarship.

My success kindled a fire in me to be one of the best in the world. I even dared to dream of being an olympian someday. This school was one of the best sprint schools in the country, with a rich tradition of graduating many great former olympians. So how could I pass up the opportunity?

My vision was very narrow-minded. It only focused on what I was going to do and what I was going to gain. Even though I was a Christian, God was in the rearview mirror. Who knows where my career would have taken me. I acknowledged that He had done a great thing in getting me where I was going, but I was at the center of the purpose. But thank God that He looks at our lives with a wider—much wider—lens.

To make a long story short, I suffered a slight tear in my left hamstring before the season started in holiday training. I still tried to compete, and only made matters worse. After going through an emotional roller coaster after the murder of my cousin Ennis, I fell into a pit of depression that seemed to have no end. I was angry with God. I felt that He had mocked me for some reason. He had given me all these things to take advantage of my opportunities and yet for some reason, here I was—alone and immobile.

I finally collected myself and began to rehabilitate. This is what later sparked my interest to pursue physical therapy. I got stronger, my flexibility returned, and I dedicated my outdoor season to Ennis in hopes that I would find a new purpose in competing. But my body never fully rebounded the way I wanted it to, making it harder and more difficult to keep up with the elite healthy athletes. My season officially (spiritually) came to an abrupt end at our first home track meet when I competed in the 400 meter hurdles.

I remember it well. I came off the turn even with the pack, feeling good, no fatigue in my body. Just when I was about to start driving down the track, I felt this gust of wind pushing me backward. Everyone flew past me, and I finished somewhere between sixth and eighth. I was dejected and confused. Looking back now, I realize that it was the hand of God, literally pushing me back. God told me that this was not the way He wanted to use me.

Now fast-forward a few years: I'm married, living in Miami, Florida, with my wife and oldest daughter. I distinctly heard God tell me that He had something for me, but that the opportunity was not in Miami. Right around the same time, my wife had recently made a visit to some friends in Atlanta, Georgia, and fell in love with the city. We immediately started praying about what to do and were led to move to Georgia. I got a great job working as a physical therapist in geriatrics and was promoted to a training position traveling across the southeast region mentoring other therapists and implementing programs for a large company. I remember thinking, "This had to be what God had planned for me, right?" Wrong!

In 2010 I finally got the vision for His purpose. I was in church one Sunday, and the bishop was preaching on God's plan for our lives. He asked the congregation if anyone had actually asked God what He wanted them to do. I realized that up to that point, I had not. So I began praying, and all of a sudden, it happened. God spoke to me. He told me to write a book.

I'd like to say that I immediately said OK and got up from my chair and headed home to begin writing, but I didn't. Actually, I asked God again to see if He was sure of what He was asking for. Maybe He said, "Klackston, I want you to write a book." Maybe it was someone else sitting behind me. He spoke again. I heard Him loud and clear this time. He told me to write a love

> "I now promote you to the position of a healer. You will heal people with both your words as a writer and your hands as a therapist."

story for young adults and mix it with all the elements of science fiction/action movies that I adored. It was to be a gift to young people about the value of accountability and the power of love. I started to sketch out the plot right there in church on the back of the church handout.

Three months and ninety-nine thousand words later the Star-Crossed Saga was born, and my career as a writer began.

But was it *the* purpose? To just write a book? It was a piece of the purpose. It was the means, but not the end. Star-Crossed was initially published in September of 2011, and God later confirmed the purpose in October of that year. Again at church, God spoke to me saying, "I now promote you to the position of a healer. You will heal people with both your words as a writer and your hands as a therapist."

That's when I started to work on both a health book (this one) and a Christian adventure series. Both are meant to inspire and encourage people through their not-so-desirable circumstances. I want to let people know that you do not have to be a victim of your own depraved thinking. You can overcome and inspire others to do the same. So my purpose is to help others to receive healing—healing of the mind, spirit, and body.

Big Takeaway: If...

1. God has a plan, then...

2. He has a purpose for it, and...

3. He has the power for that purpose to be fulfilled, and...

4. All He wants is the praise in the end.[1]

COSBY'S CORNER
To Build a Fire

Have you ever tried to build a fire in the snow? Starting a fire is hard enough on its own, much less doing it in harsh conditions of cold and snow. It's wet, damp, and breezy, providing us with everything that is essential for failure, no matter how skilled you may think you are. But that's what most of us do, isn't it? We continue to press on, building upon our past experiences to establish truth no matter how blatantly obvious it is that we are sinking, drowning in our own stubbornness and inclination to continue down paths of letdown.

Have you ever read the story *To Build a Fire* by Jack London? This short, but very beautifully written, story tells the tale of a man who is afoot, and breaks through the river ice and becomes drenched in water. As he freezes, he attempts to build a fire, rather than look for shelter from the cold. With the exception of a wolf-dog, he is alone. His faithful companion waits, sits, and watches as this man experiences failure after failure until he ultimately dies of ignorance and unremitting cold. Ironically and instinctively, the wolf-dog turns and trots up the trail in the direction of a camp, where it finds other food and fire providers.

To me, the wolf-dog represents God (and His grace), and the man is us when we are determined to do things our way rather than asking for His guidance.

It's a classic theme of man versus nature. But the nature here has a dual meaning: the power of nature and man's propensity to do things on his own, despite the incessant probability of failure. I wonder what his purpose was for building the fire. Understandably so, his first instinct was probably just to keep warm, but imagine if he had changed his focus. If he had been able to redirect all his energy toward what was really important, he may have decided that it was more expedient to find shelter in order to survive. Instead he kept working at what he thought was the best course of action: making the fire.

Do you know the definition of insanity? Continuing to do the same thing over and over, exactly the same way, and expecting different results. Are you the man trying to build a fire in the midst of a cold storm, praying that God will take your efforts and turn them into a scorching furnace, because you have yet to humble yourself to His will for your life? I would never go as far as trying to call you insane or even to compare you to the man from this story. But let's face it, anyone who continually comes up short in his efforts to do anything, with less than stellar results, deserves to have the spotlight pointed in his direction a time or two.

If you are that man and have the courage to say so, come in from the cold. Sit by the fire, take a sip of some hot cocoa, and allow God to create the ideal conditions for all-out success in your endeavors. You will not only find rest, but I also guarantee the chances of frostbite will be extremely lessened, and the outcomes will be far more comfortable. Then maybe that wolf-dog that keeps laughing at you from the corner can step in and lead you to sanctuary. I'm just saying...

■■■

Open Your Spirit to God's Plan

Typically, most folks run their lives from scripted daily routines. Wake up, take the kids to school, go to work, pick up the kids, prepare dinner, sleep, and repeat. Within all of those tasks there is more than enough opportunity for other events to take place that throw the routine way out of *whack*. Most likely, those things are more frequent than we would like for them to be. Once this happens, stress is injected back into the equation, and we have one of two options: handle it or let it handle us.

This is where most of us lose the battle. We try our best to make the right decisions, and end up chasing our tails like senseless pups. You may win one or two battles, but the war is far from over, and the small bouts of victory seldom provide the clarity that is necessary to remove stress from your life.

It is never the stress that is the problem; it is the reaction to the stress that makes the difference between peace of mind and all-out mental and physical lunacy. The yokes we take upon ourselves become heavier and heavier, consuming us like a raging fire. Our goals in life become skewed, vanishing right before our eyes, leaving some with a lacking sense of self-worth or purpose. We have become so consumed with our own visions of grandeur (that most often are unrealistic and self-serving) that the inevitable outcome of missing the mark drains the psyche and throws people into a spiral of clouded judgment.

The polarized lenses that people wear when measuring themselves against the superstars and political heroes of the world add cement blocks of unnecessary weight on their shoulders, causing them to no longer appreciate the things they do have. A burden is added to the cycle of stress that makes it harder to breathe, choking the air from the promises of possibility that come with everyday life. This should not be!

God's plans hold much more promise than anything we can think or imagine. In Jeremiah 29:11 God pleads with us to understand and trust His plans when He says, "For I know the plans that I have for you...plans for peace and not for evil, to give

> Can you really live by God's instruction and direction, outside of knowing what the future will hold?

you a future and a hope." How amazing is that? An eternal God who sits on high and looks down low upon man is not just making a powerful statement—*He is declaring that there is an irrevocable plan that He has set in motion for each one of us.* There is no mentioning that the plan is in flux, under construction, or being developed. No! God is saying that He has already determined a plan for your life. No longer do you have to burden yourself with crowding the closet of your mental thoughts with plan A and B. You can walk in faith, trust, and peace.

- *Faith*: that God is able to do what He says He can do.

- *Trust*: that your plan is special and that you have a purpose established in God.

- *Peace*: that the plan He has for you is wonderful, just as precious as His plan for the next person.

God is not a respecter of persons. He values each one of us, regarding us as His favorite child. Therefore you can walk boldly to the throne of grace and ask God to lead you. All you have to do is ask God what it is and listen to His voice. But be warned: it may involve shedding the shackles of the world and walking in the freedom that God has to offer those who can rest in the will of God. You must ask yourself if this is a step that you are truly willing to take, or if you are convinced that going in another direction of uncertainty is worth it. Can you really live by God's instruction and direction, outside of knowing what the future will hold?

God knows the plans He has for you, and it is up to you to trust that His plan is more amazing, more miraculous, and more splendid than what you believed was possible.

But it's not just about hearing what God says to you and then lying around doing absolutely nothing. God challenges you to *put the plan into action.* In Luke 14:31 Jesus speaks to the people saying, "Or what king, going to wage war against another king, does not sit down first and take counsel whether he is able with ten thousand to meet him who comes against him with twenty thousand?" The choice determines the path, but the outcome is founded on the plan that you set in motion. God respects prudent planning. Once you rest in God and He gives you the vision, creating and following a plan is critical to the degree of success. There will be challenges, struggles, and maybe even what seems like insurmountable odds placed before you, but you can overcome them in the end if your plans are in alignment with God's.

What plans do you have for the next five minutes, the next week, year, or ten years? Is God involved in these plans? If not, you need to reconsider how far you can go alone. Realize the plan for your life. Acknowledge that you have the power to take control of that plan. Assess what is necessary in order to achieve victory, and then act on it and be convinced that God will be the difference maker of your level of success.

> There will be challenges, struggles, and maybe even what seems like insurmountable odds placed before you, but you can overcome them in the end if your plans are in alignment with God's.

Submit Your Body to a Plan for Success

Research supporting the benefit of creating a regimen or routine of exercise and diet in making the difference toward life-long changes is somewhat sparse, but an article in the *Journal of the American Dietetic Association* did just that. The article, "A Structured Diet and Exercise Program Promotes Favorable Changes in Weight Loss, Body Composition, and Weight Maintenance," followed ninety obese and apparently healthy women over a ten-week university-based weight loss trial. Seventy-seven women from this sample also completed an additional twenty-four-week weight maintenance phase.

The researchers wanted to determine whether adherence to a meal-replacement-based diet program (MRP) with encouragement to increase physical activity was more effective than following a more structured meal-plan-based diet with a supervised exercise program (SDE).[2]

My favorite outcomes were used to assess results: Primary outcome measures included energy intake, physical activity, body mass, body composition, and waist and hip circumferences. Secondary outcome measures included diet quality; resting energy expenditure; markers of cardiovascular and muscular fitness; serum lipids, glucose, and insulin levels; and psychosocial assessments. These were taken at baseline and intermittently throughout the cycle of the study, including the additional twenty-four-week phase. The researchers concluded that in sedentary and obese women a more structured meal plan–based diet with a supervised exercise program appears to be more efficacious in promoting and maintaining weight loss and improvements as compared to a meal-replacement-based diet program that accompanied mere exercise encouragement.[3]

This proves two things:

1. Structured meal plan–based diets can produce better results than meal replacement ones.

2. Supervised exercise programs are obviously more powerful than unsupervised ones in producing the results you are looking for.

Therefore, the plan of attack concerning your health, your wellness, and your fitness needs to be simple. The findings of this study echoes the sentiments I wrote about earlier in the spiritual portion of the chapter:

- Plan—structure both meals and workout routines that best fit your fitness goals.

- Purpose—there must be a concise purpose or methodology to the madness. You can't just flail away at it and hope to randomly produce the results you are looking for.

- Power—you must tap into something greater than yourself. This cannot be just about you. Is the condition of your health important enough to you to create a sense of urgency in your life? Are you ready to positively affect the lives of the ones around you who rely on you to set the example— your kids, your spouse, family, and friends?

- Praise—give yourself a chance to bask in your accomplishments. Celebrate a little. A good pat on the back every now and then for meeting milestones such as ten-, twenty-, thirty-, and fifty-pound weight losses are huge. Don't downplay them for a moment. Every little bit counts toward you paying dividends for your future.

Chapter 9

BUDDY UP

H OW ABOUT BUDDYING up? Have you done it yet? Made a friend at the gym? Come on, you can do it. Remember how it was the first day your mom and dad dropped you off at kindergarten and you made your first new friend? I know, I know. It was a scary situation back then and it still is now. All those people running around, minding their own business. Some have friends already, while others just seem to have the meanest looks on their faces. You wonder why they even come to the gym looking like that if they can't be happy. Isn't exercise supposed to help you relieve stress? Many people act like they are miserable.

This should not be the case and it doesn't have to be. The road to ultimate health and wellness is paved with enough road blocks that can send you corkscrewing off the road onto the unbeaten path. So why make it that much harder by *not* taking someone along for the journey?

Set Your Mind on Sharing the Journey

They say that no man is an island, and man, is that the truth! Do you know how hard it would have been to try and build the Great Wall of China, the Statue of Liberty, the Great Pyramids, or even the fabulous city of Rome with just the work of one set of hands? It takes many people, hand-over-hand efforts pulling and lifting to fabricate, reshape, and erect a spectacle fit for the world to see. Wait a minute, doesn't that sound familiar? It kind of sounds like you, right? Something the whole world can see? But not for the benefit of superficiality, or rubbing it in the face of some long-lost love who needs to regret the day he or she walked away from you (*although I do feel you on that one, trust me*). No, this is for the glory of God. He wants you to come out of the old self and chip away at the uneven lines of despair, fill in the cracks of past failures, smooth out the rough patches of agony, and sculpt out new hope from old destitution.

> An accountability partner, someone who is in it with you for the long haul and can motivate you to stay the course, is more than a fashionable commodity; it is a necessary element to making sustainable, effective, long-term changes.

It can and will happen, but you are going to need some help along the way. Why, you ask? Well, because any journey is best taken in fellowship. Meriwether Lewis and William Clark left St. Louis in 1804 to find a water route to the Pacific, and in the end mapped out the extensive blueprint of the Rocky Mountains. Jacques Cousteau had a great team of navigators and crewmen when he studied all forms of life in the great oceans of the world. Neil Armstrong took the first steps on the moon from the Apollo 11, but he needed the two talented pilots Michael Collins and Buzz Aldrin to safely navigate space and land safely back on Earth.

You too need *not* to go the journey alone. You are primed and ready for a change in your life that will encompass a great many things. You need to eat better, be more active, set goals, and think more positively. Along the way there may be moments where you get derailed and want to quit, go back to the old way of doing things because it is easier, more comfortable. An accountability partner, someone who is in it with you, for the long haul and can motivate you to stay the course is more than a fashionable commodity; it is a necessary element to making sustainable, effective, long-term changes that you can build upon daily and meet the expectations that you *will* set for yourself—today.

COSBY'S CORNER
Any Two Will Do? Not Necessarily

As pertaining to buddying up for extra accountability and motivation, you have to keep one thing in mind: you have to choose the right person. I'm sorry to say it, but it is so true. You are judged by the company you keep, even in the fitness world. You are not judged by others per se, but by yourself. You are your biggest critic.

You know why you work out, when you work out, where you work out, and who you choose to work out with. If you've ever had a chance to work out with someone other than your best friend, say a personal trainer, physical therapist, or spin instructor, you know that the experience can be no joke. At times during the session you could feel like flat out giving up. But that is good! You should feel like that.

Working out is serious business because your body doesn't normally trend toward the path of pain, fatigue, and discomfort. Most bouts of exercise entail all three, if you are doing it correctly. Don't get me wrong, there are limitations to how hard you should work out and the amount of burn you should feel, but again you have to be your toughest critic.

Maybe you're honestly not a good gauge of what you should feel like. OK, here's a suggestion: If you are able to walk out of the gym feeling exactly the same way you felt when you came in, you didn't work hard enough. Therefore, if you are buddying up with someone who is not pushing you, encouraging you to do one more set, one more repetition, or walk that extra minute and a half, you might need to change. And don't get mad because you feel that person is nagging you. You need it! Friends don't let friends drink and drive. The same thing goes for working out. Friends don't let friends drink and glide.

- *Drink*: sipping on water in the shade or sitting on the bench resting for long periods of time when you should be working up a sweat

- *Glide*: simply gliding through the workout routine without wincing one bit or cringing because your muscles are burning

Your buddy needs to motivate you to stay diligent and focused. Even if the two of you look like circus elephants doing those tricks with the ringmaster, it's all good, folks. So what! Not everybody in the gym needs to look like Schwarzenegger (the old one from *Conan*) or Jillian Michaels. What really matters is that you do your absolute best.

Work with what you have, and work within your limits. Set boundaries for heart rate, respiratory rate, sets, and repetitions. Try to hug those standards as close as possible during your sessions so that you will excel and meet higher goals each and every week you go to the gym. Add more weight, more reps, more sets, walk longer, and run faster.

Picking the right workout buddy can elevate your personal bests within no time, but you have to make the right decision of who is going to go with you.

Also pick someone who is pretty close to your style of training and is working toward achieving similar goals. Matching up a 5k runner with a body builder in the gym makes absolutely no sense at all. The same goes for you. If you are a first timer, why not start off with a personal trainer to familiarize yourself with the gym? Ask the trainer to slowly break you in over a few weeks so that you do not get too discouraged too soon. Then, after a few weeks, find a person who you feel is going to push you just as much as you will push him or her back. That way, as iron sharpens iron, one hand washes another, and both of you become that support system that will have you on your way to the mall to try on those skinny jeans.

Remember, you have a choice of what this workout thing can and will look like. Playing around in the gym going through the motions is just like a dog chasing its tail. It may feel as though it's getting closer every time, but in the end, you and I both know it accomplished only one thing: it got dizzy. I'm just saying . . .

■■■

Biblical Buddy System Examples

The Bible is full of stories highlighting the power of the *buddy system*: Paul and Barnabas, David and Jonathan, Elijah and Elisha, Moses and Aaron, Joshua and Caleb, and Mary and Martha. These people performed amazing acts of faith and restitution, but consider this simple principle: They had someone at their side to support them when they got weak, discouraged, or needed encouragement. Who knows where they would have ended up had it not been for their partnership?

God understands the value of having companionship on life's great journeys. If it were not so, we would never have had the examples of these people's lives placed before us. I challenge you to read just a few excerpts from the Bible about the people mentioned above, then tell me if you think that they would have

> There will be no communion, cooperation, or success without agreement.

been able to endure through the tough times on their own. I think you'll find that it was more than necessary to have someone by their side who understood their struggles in the natural world. God is always present to supply our every need including encouragement and inspiration, but He knows us all too well. He knows that we will face things in the world that will quickly detour us from the path to ultimate wellness that He needs us to be on in order to do His will.

What's even more wonderful is that God does not leave you in the midst of a struggle, even if you have someone with you. He does not expect you to rely on others to get through the rough patches under your own power. He implores us to:

• Come together

• Encourage (sharpen) one another

• Understand that He will be there in the midst of our partnership to assist us and make up the difference

Here's what God says to His people in the Bible on these topics:

> Do two people walk together, if they have not agreed?
> —Amos 3:3

> Iron sharpens iron, so a man sharpens the countenance of his friend.
> —Proverbs 27:17

> For where two or three are assembled in My name, there I am in their midst.
> —Matthew 18:20

You see, God urges us to come together and agree on what is needed to be done. There will be no communion, cooperation, or success without agreement. Your walk down this road of breaking the cycles of defeat needs to be a slow, calculated trot. One that is supported by a friend, mentor, and partner or buddy who can equally support you and receive the backing that you have to offer. You are there not only to receive, but to sharpen the other one.

When iron is pulled from the fire and begins to take form, it is clanged against itself under pressure and force. Each piece sharpens the other, smoothing out the lumps, straightening the dents, and sealing away the cracks that can possibly reduce the effect of its use. You must become that iron. You must help someone else also find his or her purpose and meet their goals. Remember the lesson of giving instead of getting from the last chapter.

If the iron was perfect in the first place, there would be no reason for it to be sharpened. It happens over time and not by chance. It was *made* to be perfect. But it, just like you, needs support from an outside source. God is the great blacksmith, and He uses someone else to build, form, and mold you into the powerful tool for His workmanship.

When you come together to meet the challenge and stretch your hand toward attaining the prize of meeting your goals, God will dwell in the midst of the occasion. He will not only support you and your companion, giving you the tools to succeed, but He will make up the difference where you are not able to *deliver the goods* just yet.

It only takes the determination and a little sacrifice of the things that have held you back all this time to receive the deliverance that God holds in His hands. He will not willingly hand over the whole thing to you, but He will ration it out, bit by bit in order to keep you hungry. He wants to see you fight for what is most important, and do it while considering the needs of another. Then, once you and your buddy have achieved the victory, He will be able to be exalted.

The Buddy System at Work in Your Body

We've seen a spiritual illustration of the power we possess in teamwork, but you may be asking where the scientific manifestation of this principle is. I cite two referenced works by Dr. Thomas Plante, a PhD in psychology at Santa Clara University to support this.

The first one comes from an article from the *American Journal of Health Behavior*, which posed the question concerning the implementation of using an iPod during exercise versus going it alone or with a friend. Dr. Plante wanted to examine the role of music and social contact on exercise benefits. They (he and his researchers) took a sample of two hundred twenty-nine students and assigned them (randomly) to perform twenty minutes of exercise at 70 per-

> Music and social contact generally enhanced mood, enjoyment, and psychological functioning.

cent of their maximal heart rate across one of six conditions: biking alone with iPod or friend in a laboratory, walking alone with iPod or friend outdoors, or biking or walking alone in controlled conditions.[1]

The participants completed various objective tests/questionnaires: AD-ACL, PES, PACES, and a ten-point Likert scale to affirm momentary mood states, perceived exertion, the amount of enjoyment individuals have during an exercise, and to capture perceived stress levels during the activity, respectively. Overall, they discovered that music and social contact generally enhanced mood, enjoyment, and psychological functioning, and controlled indoor conditions resulted in a more relaxed and calm response.

The next article by Dr. Plante comes from the *Journal of Social Science*. Here he looked at the social comparison theory to examine if exercising with a research confederate posing as either *high fit* or *low fit* would increase the exertion in exercising.[2] He and his team of researchers wanted to know if the perception of exercise intensity as related to what a person expects his/her training partner to be able to do would affect that person's level or intensity of exertion.

In the study, ninety-one college students were asked to complete twenty minutes of exercise at 60–70 percent of their maximum target heart rate under these randomly assigned conditions: biking alone, biking with a high-fit, or biking with a low-fit partner. Across four standardized checklists and self-assessment questionnaires, it was concluded that participants in the high fit condition exercised harder than those in the low fit conditions.

In both studies there is an appreciable difference of results for people who train and exercise with a partner with varying conditions—whether inside or outside—than people who go it alone.

I love the second study the most because it speaks to our own competitive nature as human beings. We live to be the best, or we die trying. Our carnal nature to dominate, win, or conquer our opponent is valuable when it comes to exercise. I told you earlier that we must have something outside of ourselves to take us to the next level. Working with a buddy is the added incentive that we all need. It's not about going into something just to best the other person and shame them. It's more or less creating an environment of change that involves external motivational factors that will push you toward your goals.

The things that occur within your mind that constantly beckon you to either press forward or quit need to be stimulated or inhibited. That inspiration can come in the form of a friend who values you and respects what you are striving to accomplish. *Buddying-up* is not just a choice when it comes to health and wellness; it is a necessity that can bring forth amazing results, and supply both you and your partner with the confidence you need to reach your full potential.

Chapter 10

GET MOVING

T HROUGHOUT THIS BOOK I have introduced you to the concept of getting outside of yourself to discover the power of embracing a purpose that includes giving of yourself to others. We looked at the tools God has given us in the fruit of the Spirit, tools that will help you to overcome a "me first, me only" mind-set about the journey to health. I helped you to understand that helping others right now while you are still in the process of your own journey to health will give you even greater motivation to stay with the plan. Then I gave you important insights to show you how to listen to the voice of God to discover your own unique, specially created purpose for all you do. That purpose will include reaching outside of yourself to others.

There is so much power in dedicating yourself to something bigger than just your own personal space. We are so much more than just the amount of money we have in the bank, personal possessions, and wants and needs. When people truly make the right steps to making a difference in the world we live in, I believe they tap into a source of power greater than just that of their own. Many of these individuals are able to touch hundreds of thousands and millions of people across the globe.

You can only get back what you are willing to give out freely. There is no one-sided consequence in life. What you put out will return to you, more than you give, and greater than you give. The degree of the outcomes of our daily lives can best be predicted on the energy we put behind something.

In this chapter we will look at some specific information in each of the three areas of mind, spirit, and body that demonstrate the power both of connecting with the power of our faith in God, and of partnering with others in our own lives.

Mind or Spirit or Mind and Spirit?

There is an underlying current of discord between science and the spirit world. I'm not talking about some mindless chanting, smoke and mirror ploys, or reading of cards to find purpose and healing. I'm speaking specifically to tapping into the power of faith-driven healing, which allows

> Current research now highlights the physical benefits of having a spiritual connection with faith, religion, or spirituality.

us to walk in the freedom of health and wellness through our God-given inheritance.

Current research now highlights the physical benefits of having a spiritual connection with faith, religion, or spirituality. Some specific research comes from a conglomeration of information collected in an article of the *Journal of Athletic Training*. The objectives of the study done by lead researcher, Brian E. Udermann, PhD, were to examine if topics related to spirituality were being addressed in the curricula of athletic training programs, and to investigate whether program directors believed this to be a topic worthy of inclusion in athletic programs.[1]

The researchers searched MEDLINE from 1976 to 1999 using various key words like spirituality, religion, healing, faith, and health. The findings in related studies were nothing less than astonishing. They included:

1. Supportive evidence for linking spiritual commitment and general health. Men who believed that spiritual commitment was important trended to have lower diastolic blood pressures than those who did not.[2] This carries over into lower rates of arteriosclerotic disease in men and women,[3] longer life span,[4] and greater levels of happiness and life satisfaction.[5]

2. Scientific proof on the effect of faith and spiritual commitment on healing and recovery. Heart-transplant recipients regularly attending spiritual services and who reported having strong spiritual beliefs had better compliance with rehabilitation protocols, reported higher emotional well-being indexes, and had superior physical functioning capabilities.[6]

3. There is power in prayer. Amongst a coronary care population of 393 patients, those who randomly received daily intercessory prayer or no prayer at all from a group of nondenominational Christians, significantly differed (positively) from those not receiving prayer on six variables at discharge

form the hospital (less intubation and ventilation assist, fewer antibiotics, diuretics, cardiopulmonary arrests, episodes of congestive heart failure, and fewer cases of pneumonia).[7]

It's fascinating to me how science is now able to prove (to some degree) that there are benefits with being connected to a higher power. It's not only fascinating that they are able to but also that it's taken this long. Sure enough, the trend is slowly shifting in the favor of believers. Now we must testify to the truth of what we know.

COSBY'S CORNER
Hold On Playa

All right everyone, it's time to have a little fun. You've been good so far in this journey, trekking through the pages of this book—probably being way too serious—so we are going to kick back and laugh a little. This Cosby's Corner is a real doozy.

On *Ask the Fat Doctors*, Jamie and I used to bounce perspectives off one another each week about things that make you have to say, "Hold on, playa!" It was a term coined by a good friend of Jamie's, NFL legend Deion Sanders, to document embarrassing things people do in public. I'm going to share three Hold on playas with you that relate to this chapter.

First up, the issue of men wearing skinny jeans. I mean seriously, to me, I think there are fashion trends that need to be either discarded or revised, with a disclaimer attached. The discarded types also include wearing your pants off the edge of your butt, or wearing socks with slippers. They are both equally ridiculous. But skinny jeans are of the revised variety. Really because there are different levels of skinny jeans.

Some skinny jeans are stylish, hugging the lower leg only and giving some room in the middle, more sensitive area. Others are just an offense to the eyes.

One shudders at the thought of how some of these fellas even fit into them and have the strength to walk afterward. Furthermore, we have to consider the age groups that should be allowed to even attempt to wear them. Let's make a cut-off age for the tight-fitting ones, say, hmm, boy-band demographic.

If you are too old to make it in a boy band, then you are too old to wear tight-fitting skinny jeans. Also, if your stomach hangs over your belt, you are banned from wearing skinny jeans. I will not even attempt to elaborate on why this rule should be put into effect. Let's just leave the tight-fitting skinny jeans to the rock stars. They are on stage for a limited amount of time, they are appealing to an audience that is more into their music than their clothing preferences, and let's face it—they are rock stars. They can just about get away with doing anything. You, on the other hand, are not. Hold on playa!

Second, why do people always love to say they are big-boned when they need to lose some weight? It's funny to think that I have never heard of anyone who is skinny say that they are big-boned. First of all, from a scientific standpoint, it's not the truth. Nobody here on planet Earth is running around with a set of bones that are bigger than the average human being that predisposes you to be overweight. When I say this, I mean having excess weight. OK, what I'm trying to say is that having larger bones does not make you grow more fat.

Look at the average NBA player. Yeah, they have big bones, meaning they have bones that are longer and denser than the rest of us, but they are not all walking around with fat busting out of their uniforms.

For every person that you know who says he or she is big-boned (maybe you are included in this group), I challenge you to ask to see a baby picture of that person from the age of birth to two years. Take a good look at his or her bones and tell me if you think that they look any bigger than the average birth-to-two-year-old's bones. Surely you'll agree with me that they are just using this term to excuse their inability to get serious about losing weight. Hold on playa!

Last, who decided that it was OK to lower the bar when it comes to wearing spandex in public? It's one thing to wear whatever you want to wear to the beach. I'm from Miami, and I've been to the beach more than my fair share. Trust me when I say that there are some people who have no shame. But it's excusable because they are on the beach. I just turn my head the other way. Spandex is another story.

For some reason, people seem to think that they can wear it anywhere like it's a pair of jeans. The mall, the grocery store, and even the post office. Is any place sacred? Just because you can stuff it in the spandex, doesn't mean that it fits.

Not sure if you qualify to wear spandex? OK, then here's the official spandex test. If you can do this, then you just keep on doing your thing and wear them to your heart's desire. Put on, pull up, stretch, tug, bend, lay on the couch, hold your breath, kick, scream, or whatever you need to do to get them on and then stand perfectly still. Take in a deep breath, think of the most relaxing place on Earth and go there. You are there, all alone, not a single care in the world, and no one to say a single thing about you. Now, exhale! Look down at your feet. If you cannot see them, you have just failed. Please remove the spandex, along with any ideas of exiting the house with them on. Feel free to wear them inside your home only. That way, no one has to be extra polite with their eyes and turn away, or give you a phony smile when you make eye contact with them because they are trying to mask what they are thinking. You know what they are dying to say to you: Hold on playa!

Disclaimer: This message was not intended to offend anyone, but to motivate you to get your act together first. Then you can feel free to push the envelope a little concerning the aforementioned topics. I am Dr. Braxton A. Cosby, and I wrote it, so of course, I approve this message. I'm just saying . . .

■■■

Inspiration for Your Spirit

You will have ups and downs, struggles, moments of hitting the wall and wanting to quit—we all do at times. It will be very difficult for you to stay committed to losing weight and cleansing your mind if you and the things that you want are your only source of inspiration. But if you can tap into another degree of commitment, the material summation of wins and losses will continue to dwindle in your mind and make it so much easier to stay the course. The *natural world's* distractions will be fewer and far between. You will see only the victory waiting for you at the end of the tunnel. But this can be achieved only if you find a connection with your heavenly Father. He provides power beyond strength, joy beyond happiness, fulfillment surpassing contentment. All of these are possible when you bond with the will of God. But it must start with you making the decision to adhere to a covenant relationship.

Two passages of Scripture highlight the tone of the times that we are in right now: times of decision making, revelation, and heightened anticipation. In Matthew 11:12 Jesus spoke:

> From the days of John the Baptist until now, the kingdom of heaven has forcefully advanced, and the strong take it by force.

The kingdom of heaven is advancing. Wow! God's kingdom is in constant motion. Can you imagine this? God's kingdom has been in constant motion since Jesus spoke these words. There has not been a single off day. Angels, elders, and spirits have been doing God's work since these words were captured. There is a plan that God has enacted, and He has charged His army with duties of carrying out scripted events to set things in motion. God knows the end of a thing, just as much as He knows the beginning. Therefore, it is important for us to know that He has set the world in motion, like a spinning top, and He knows exactly the instant that it will stop turning and topple over. He has made every concession and established every regulation to make sure that His plans are fulfilled to be in exact

> There is a real chance that the kingdom may advance past you and you could miss the opportunity to tap into the power that is freely given to those who join forces—if you choose not to believe.

correlation with His written Word, the Bible. This *advancing* dictates that we must all be on our guard because just as much as there is a good kingdom advancing to the end of days, there is an evil one as well. Forceful men, both fueled by good and evil intentions, are laying hold of the kingdom.

Please understand this point: there is a real chance that the kingdom may advance past you and you could miss the opportunity to tap into the power that is freely given to those who join forces—if you choose not to believe. At your fingertips is the chance to receive authority to perform signs, miracles, and acts that glorify God while aiding you in exceeding your personal goals. No one is better than the next person, and God is not a respecter of persons. Each one of us has a reserved position in the army of God's great kingdom. We have the right to receive the gifts that He freely gives, without obligation of any kind, but we have to be willing to sacrifice our allegiance to the things of this world in order to get them.

In 2 Peter 1:10 it states:

> Therefore, brothers, diligently make your calling and election sure. For if you do these things, you will never stumble.

Peter makes a proposal to us all. He warns us to be eager in making our election and calling sure by dedicating ourselves to the principles and ideals of the Father. There is a responsibility laid before us to decide to what we are willing to entrust our souls. He says that we have been called and elected, so why would we hand over the keys to our office and position to those who would only desire to destroy us. We have been given a gift—one that we have not even had to work for—and we should honor that gift by pressing all the harder to excel at it.

When someone is elected as the president, do they not attempt to do all that is necessary to prove to the people who put them in office that they are worthy of the honor? So the same should be with us. We have been elected as children of God, soldiers for the cross, and heirs to the gifts of the kingdom. Therefore victory is ours in everything that we do as long as we are willing to follow the guidance of God and give Him praise for what He does in our lives.

Our thoughts, our habits, and the ritualistic way of thinking that has constructed our persona up to this point may need to be discarded. We just may need to relinquish our old doctrine and take on a new one that will redefine who we consider ourselves to be. It will be more about *whose* we are than *who* we are. If we can get with the movement, the spiritual movement of God, we will see His good and perfect will for our lives. We will be able to more importantly affect the lives of others. Then the kingdom will continue to grow and prosper in the way God intended it to. The power to both do and be everything we ever wanted is already available to us. We need only make the choice. We are called to be so much more than what we are, but we fail to do greater things because we believe so little. In order to fully appreciate what we are called to do, we must build our relationship with Him.

> Victory is ours in everything that we do as long as we are willing to follow the guidance of God and give Him praise for what He does in our lives.

The Spirit Connection With Your Body

The field of complementary medicine is catching on fast to the efficacy of healing and the use of nonmedicinal approaches to wellness. There have been numerous studies to prove it, more than three hundred fifty to be exact. These studies of physical health used religious and spiritual variables and found that there are correlations associated with better health outcomes.[8] These studies deal with disorders of the mind (soul) such as depression, anxiety, alcoholism, cigarette smoking and other forms of substance abuse, and suicide.

- *Depression*: Did you know that 6–10 percent of the population experiences or will experience significant depression during their lifetime?[9] That's a little fewer than 700 million people. One study of 177 persons (aged 55–89 years) examined the effects of self-reported religious salience on the incidence and course of depression over one year. Religious salience was associated with less risk of depression and strongly associated with recovery from depression among those individuals that reported being depressed at the beginning of the study. It was especially prevalent in those in poor physical health.[10]

- *Anxiety*: There is a strong association between people reporting to have less anxiety and being involved in religion. Scientists examined the relationship between the spiritual well-being of 114 adults newly diagnosed with cancer; patients with high levels of spiritual well-being had lower levels of anxiety regardless of sex, age, marital status, diagnosis, group participation, or time since diagnosis.[11]

• *Substance abuse*: Religious persons are less likely to use or abuse alcohol and other drugs. A review of twenty published studies found that religious involvement was associated with less substance abuse, with the measure of religious involvement defined as membership, active participation, religious upbringing, or self-reported religious salience.[12]

• *Suicide*: Apparently there is an inverse relationship between religious involvement and suicide. Self-reported religiosity and attendance at religious services have been shown to be inversely associated with suicidal ideation.[13]

Those are just some of the positive influences religion has on the mental well-being of individuals. Never mind the numerous studies on the positive effects of having a spiritual relationship or religious connection with God with conditions of the body: hypertension, cardiovascular disease, exercise, and mortality. Forming a spiritual connection isn't just for adults. It's beneficial for children and adolescents as well. Development of this relationship yields its best results when introduced early on. Children born into religiously involved families learn healthy behaviors, but also view their religious and spiritual relationships as sources of hope, comfort, and support.[14]

In addition, religious and spiritual practices (for example meditation, prayer, and worship) can encourage other positive emotions such as love, contentment, and forgiveness, limiting negative emotions such as hostility. From a scientific level, positive emotions can limit the activation of the sympathetic branch of the autonomic nervous system and the hypothalamic-pituitary adrenal axis allowing a decreased release of stress hormones such as norepinephrine and cortisol (shown to be responsible for weight gain). This response can decrease blood pressure, heart rate, and oxygen consumption, leading to better health.[15] In fact, religiously involved persons have enhanced immune function when compared to uninvolved persons.[16]

Health-Related Quality of Life (HRQOL)

Last, and this is huge, the term I want to share with you is *health-related quality of life*. It refers to the distinct physical, psychological, social, and spiritual domains of health that are influenced by a person's experiences, beliefs, expectations, and perceptions.[17] Studies show that there is a high correlation between religious involvement and spiritual well-being with high levels of HRQOL in persons with cancer, HIV disease,[18] heart disease,[19] limb amputation, and spinal cord injury.[20] Ironically, this direct relationship between spirituality

> Positive emotions can limit the activation of the sympathetic branch of the autonomic nervous system and the hypothalamic-pituitary adrenalaxis allowing a decreased release of stress hormones such as norepinephrine and cortisol (shown to be responsible for weight gain).

and HRQOL persists regardless of declines in physical functioning.[21]

In general, the data clearly shows that there is a definite correspondence between spirituality and healthy living. There is indeed power, strength, authority, and wellness that affect our mental and physical symptoms, as well as positively influencing our degree of quality of life.

Eat Less, Move More

This chapter has been filled with evidence that a decision to change—in your mind, spirit, or body is going to require movement—moving forward toward your goal of wellness. I have something that is going to get you started on your road to fitness. Forget all the complicated programs out there, and remember four words: *eat less* and *move more*. This is going to be our campaign for the next thirty days. Consider this book, especially this section, as a jump start on the life-changing path ahead of you.

> People have been lulled to sleep, feeling as though conceiving the idea of being healthy and fit is reserved for an elite few.

"So what is the Eat Less, Move More Campaign?" you ask. It's simple. It's my attempt at getting you in shape, and not just physical shape, but also mental shape. This is a plan to awaken your inner hero—the inner victor!

I believe that people have been lulled to sleep, feeling as though conceiving the idea of being healthy and fit is reserved for an elite few. I believe that is entirely not true. Back in 2014 I coordinated a twelve-week boot camp in Atlanta where we implemented Eat Less, Move More and met only once a week for one bout of exercise utilizing the Chachersize for Men routine. These fifteen to twenty individuals lost more than a combined one hundred pounds. So I know it works. Remember: each one of us has a purpose, and fulfilling that purpose starts with being physically ready to perform. But before you can be physically ready, you need to be mentally prepared.

People are losing the fight against the diseases of excess weight; but the battle starts in the space between your ears. All of those convoluted diets, exercise programs, and fitness fads are doing some good for a select few, but the majority of the population is just getting tired. The Eat Less, Move More Campaign is an attempt at calibrating your mind. If you can follow the campaign as closely as possible to my recommendations, I believe that over time you will develop a stronger will to take hold of your health.

This is a two-part campaign, requiring your personal dedication.

1. Part one—eat less. Take your normal portions of food, all three meals, and cut them in half. Save it for later, give it away, whatever. But don't eat the same portion any longer.

2. Part two—move more. Purchase a pedometer and track the amount of steps you take a day. Now try to double that over the next twenty-nine days.

Why Will It Work?

This challenge will work for you because you've never done it before. You need to change the way you think and destroy old habits. Stacking that plate is hurting you, and trying difficult exercise programs without embracing change (slowly) is discouraging you. This will retrain both your mind and body gradually.

Over the next thirty days I am asking you to stand with me and make a change in your life. Don't put this off until tomorrow or next week. Make the choice to live today. Don't do it just for your family and friends, but do it for yourself.

Once you complete the thirty days, feel free to take it to the next level. Make small gains first by finishing whatever you start. The time is now! You've heard my pep talk. What are you waiting for? Get moving!

Chapter 11

THERE ARE NO PERFECT CIRCUMSTANCES

Wouldn't it be nice if everything was served up to us on a silver platter? I mean, we would love nothing more than to just snap our fingers and find someone right there to cater to our every need at the drop of a hat. No work, no cares, no worries, no nothing. Life would be just splendid. We'd all have perfect spouses and kids, fantastic jobs (work from home making six figures), and the bodies of gods and goddesses. Is anyone up for something similar to this? Sure you are. But unfortunately, life is about work. Some people have to put in more effort than others to get the things they want and need. In the end, there is some degree of effort that needs to be actualized for each of us.

To that extent, I wish that living healthy was easy. I will not lie to you and say that it is, because it is not. Everything around us is a setup to fail. Grocery stores place all the necessary items in the back of the store and force you to walk past all the buy-one-get-one-free items (most of which are sugar depots). Fast-food restaurants are on just about every corner, and the food is not just fast, it's also cheap. Five to six bucks gets you a meal, and the fast-food chicken restaurants can feed an entire family on just ten dollars. What budget- and time-constrained family is not going to jump all over that? Less energy, less money, and the kids love it.

Get in the Right Frame of Mind

I want you to try and motivate you for a moment. There is a way to stay focused, even amongst the distractions of the outside, fat-filled world. But first you have to do something for me. Raise your right hand and repeat after me: "I am overweight, overworked, mentally strained, and spiritually depleted." Pick one of those, or all of them if it fits. Now, keeping it raised say this: "I am responsible for my state, right now, and will be responsible going forward. Any excuse I have about not making a change is *my* excuse, and I am fully accountable to it." Great! Now we are ready.

> You think that the mind is the battleground for overcoming your struggles and the key to breaking the cycles of defeat. You're wrong, my friend! It's your body.

I want you to try and imagine for a moment that you have the ability to split yourself in half. One half is your body, and the other half is your mind. Your body makes its own decisions—what to eat, what to wear, how much exercise to do, and even what essential bodily functions to perform and monitor. Your mind is only responsible for two things—determining what is good for you and what is bad.

The two halves are in constant conflict with one another. Your mind doesn't want you to be unhealthy. It only wants you to be happy, possessing the ability to move, breathe, and be productive. You think that the mind is the battleground for overcoming your struggles and the key to breaking the cycles of defeat. You're wrong, my friend! It's your body. Your body is the alpha dog. It is an efficient machine that is constantly making sophisticated calculations and decisions. The minute you put anything into your body, or perform one repetition of exercise, proclaim one positive or negative thing about yourself, your body makes the smallest appreciable change toward one thing: homeostasis (the body's tendency to maintain a stable, relatively constant condition of properties). It wants to survive, and be good at it.

Your body likes the way you are right now. It has gotten used to managing it that way. It has you on a schedule. Food in, break it down, store the excess, and remove the waste. It has expectations of what each day entails. Shake up the schedule a little bit and the body attempts to respond the best way it can to the given situation. Provide a stress to the system—like intense aerobic exercise that really challenges you—it will make changes instantly in preparation for the next bout. Slack off the next day, week, or month, and the body goes right back to where it was previously, low expectations and all. It will even begin to hold on to things like fat if it thinks that you will need it later.

Think of it this way. If I told you that your job was going to cut your wages for the next three months and you had two months to prepare, what would you do? Hopefully, you'd begin to save a little and then be a bit more frugal with your spending over the next three months so that you can survive. That's what the body does with fat storage. Your body has no clue when the flow of food will cease, so it continues to hold on to fat as a safety net. When you starve yourself and do not eat, you ask your body to do exactly what you would do if your money flow suddenly dwindled. If you eat constantly throughout the day (only the right foods, three meals, plus two to three healthy snacks) you train your body to release fat.

The same can be said about exercise. Your body has two muscle types—fast- and slow-twitch muscles. There is a percentage of each one in us based on genetics and lifestyle. You cannot ever become entirely one or the other. If you are a sedentary person, your body has a higher number of fast-twitch muscle fibers, which help you explode quickly for limited amounts of time before you get fatigued. If you are very active, then you probably have more slow-twitch fibers, and you can sustain high-level bouts of activity over time. Your body hits a transitional *switch* when exposed to increased or decreased activity concerning these fiber types.

That's why exercise hurts at first, but then gets progressively better over time if you hang in there. You begin to develop the right kind of muscle fibers for the job at hand. But this takes effort and energy for your body to keep up. It'd rather spend the majority of its time managing the essential organs of the body (heart, lungs, skin, and so forth) rather than repairing smooth muscle. That throws off its efficiency.

> Some days will be harder than others. Stay the course. You have to decide to do it now. Your body will listen and respond.

You are fighting your body's tendency to maintain its homeostatic environment. My body likes me being slim. I'm very predictable that way. If I put on a lot of weight unexpectedly, it would have a hard time adjusting. The same is true with you. If you are overweight, your body is happy that way.

Inject a little exercise and diet, and your body is going to talk to you. It's going to tell you that you need to do what you used to because it is a selfish machine. It's sort of like an accountant who gets frustrated because you fail to turn in the accurate numbers when filing your taxes.

You think it's your mind fighting you, but believe me, folks, it's your body. You have the chance to turn things around by controlling your mind and not believing that you are defeated. You can make a difference in your health. It starts the moment you decide to change things around, to work them in your favor. There will not be any perfect circumstances for you. Some days will be harder than others. Stay the course. You have to decide to do it now. Your body will listen and respond. All you have to do is ignore it when it talks back.

COSBY'S CORNER
The Difference Between Five-Star and Five Stars

There is a big discrepancy in this world between effort and outcomes. Some people define working out as strenuous bouts of exercise that deplete the living life-force out of you and make you dread going back to the gym the next day. While others simply believe that breaking a sweat is the mark or definition of true weight-loss championing. I believe that the truth lies somewhere in the middle. As a matter of fact, one of my mentors used to say that there are three sides to every story—yours, mine, and the truth. Unfortunately, the disparity between the two opinions concerning exercise holds the all-important prize: the outcome.

When I was a child, my mother decided to take the family on a European tour via bus. We were set to travel from one country to the next, taking in the beautiful sights and sounds of each destination.

I can recall her talking to my grandmother and describing what the travel detailed about each of the hotels we were going to stay at during our travels. Plus, we would stay in luxurious and extravagant four- and five-star hotels that would make any American salivate at the mouth. Again, as a child I had no frame of reference for the rating. My mother explained that four to five stars meant something very nice was in store for us. I imagined it to be something really sweet like the fancy hotels and restaurants in New York City. Our entire family bought it, especially because the price was a real steal. So we were set, right, made in the shade? This is Cosby's Corner, folks! So needless to say, boy was I and everyone else on the trip very wrong.

What was defined as five stars in Europe was probably more like a two-star dig in the United States. I'd liken it to eating a can of Spam versus filet mignon. That was an overshoot. Maybe it was more like a nice Philly cheesesteak sandwich.

Each place we bounced to across Europe set a hilarious standard for the next one. By the time the trip was over, all we could do was laugh our way through Europe. I actually began to anticipate arriving at the next five-star crash site, just to see if it was worse than the previous one. Most times it didn't disappoint. I remember kissing the ground at the airport when we got back to Miami. There's a distinct difference between five-star and five stars.

My experience was kind of like what people perceive in their minds as a great workout when they go to the gym. Some people are present, going through the motions and putting forth an effort, while others are really killing it—making the shorts on their backsides rip from their skin or saturate with so much sweat you grimace at the thought of using the machine after they are through with it.

Still others are hitting the sweet spot. Their workouts add just enough resistance to stress their muscles and provide the perfect degree of difficulty to challenge their cardiovascular capability. They see results on a monthly, if not weekly basis.

I don't want to take away from the second group, which is probably the five-star varieties. But truly, the four-star folks are probably the level where most people want to be.

Examine yourself just a little closer when you go to the gym. Look around, take in the sights. Are you really brave enough to compare yourself to the Ritz Carltons and the Caesar's Palaces of the world? Or are you just a European version of the real thing? I'm just saying...

■■■

Inject Some Spirit Energy

Are you feeling drained physically, emotionally, and mentally? Does it seem like even talking about the idea of exercise sucks the life right out of you? You are not alone. A lot of people tell me that they feel this way. Busy schedules and life changes exist, and they are real. In order to tend to these obligations, you need to have energy. Beyond the right balance of diet and exercise, you need something else. You must inject the Spirit of God into the equation if you are to possess sustainable strength for the journey. You have to accept the idea that God is able to give this to you freely. He can ignite the torch of the spirit of strength in you. He did it for Samson. In Judges 15:14–16, it says:

> He came to Lehi, and the Philistines shouted as they approached him. Then the Spirit of the LORD came mightily upon him. The ropes on his arms became like burned flax and the ties on his hands dissolved. Then he found a fresh jawbone of a donkey, reached out his hand and took it, and with it struck down a thousand men. Samson said,
>
> "With a jawbone of a donkey,
>   heaps upon heaps.
> With a jawbone of a donkey
>   I have slain a thousand men."

Yes, with a donkey's jawbone, folks. Are you kidding me? That had to be nothing but God right there. It says that the Spirit of God came powerfully on Samson. He broke free from his restraints and picked up the weapon of his choosing to slay a thousand men.

> You must inject the Spirit of God into the equation if you are to possess sustainable strength for the journey.

If God can give Samson that type of power, imagine what He can do for you. All you're asking is for Him to help you take on the treadmill for thirty minutes. That type of Samson power is nice to have, but you only require an ounce of it to get through your daily routines. You don't have to be a powerful Nazarite to pull off these feats of bravery. All you have to do is call on God and let the One who knows all about your struggles help you in the best way that He sees fit. He could have given Samson a machine gun. He could have dropped it right out of heaven, but He didn't. He gave him only what was necessary to get the job done. No matter your background, health, and past limitations, God can give you the victory.

He also knows precisely how to meet us where we are. None of our present circumstances excuse us from facing the challenge set before us. We have the choice to either change or remain the same.

> All you have to do is call on God and let the One who knows all about your struggles help you in the best way that He sees fit.

Paul wrote the majority of the New Testament, and it wasn't without persecution. But the road to his brilliant future in Christ was not paved with roses. God sought after him. Within all of Paul's faults, failures, and offenses against God, there was a hope instilled inside of him that was coated in a shiny veil of deliverance.

Paul was at first named Saul. On the road to Damascus, God cried out to him, "Saul, Saul, why do you persecute Me?" (Acts 9:4). Do you know what made the difference in Paul's conversion? He believed. He believed that he was hearing the voice of a God who was able to give Him the strength to do more than he imagined. He knew God was able to take him to a level that he never conceived within himself to be possible. His strength came from the fact that he was destined to be used for a greater purpose than that of the self-made agenda that he was running after. That purpose fortified his dedication to make changes in his life that would effectually change the lives of others someday. It wasn't about excuses or poor timing. Paul chose the time to be just right.

Time and time again, God meets us right where we are. Rather than asking us to do something supernatural, He prepares the way, choosing to perform something spectacular inside of us. Why do we constantly try the opposite with Him? We ask for supernatural events from God to prove who He is, and then we'd like to think that we'll be able to get our act together, fully knowing that all we'd do is wait again for some other miracle before we do what we need to do and what we can do. Kill the excuses, make the right decision, and pray to God for the ability to overcome your circumstances and accomplish the goals that lie before you. Go for the low hanging fruit that is right at your fingertips. You no longer have to ask someone else to do the picking. It's your time, right now.

Give Your Body the Correct Technique

Good form and technique during an exercise session are not just safe, but essential for obtaining maximal results. The idea that you can just go to the gym and lumber through each repetition and set, working up a sweat and seeing the outcomes you desire concerning strength gains and losing weight is somewhat farfetched. Will you see some changes at the physical level by just changing your routine and actively engaging in a routine outside of just being a couch

> Kill the excuses, make the right decision, and pray to God for the ability to overcome your circumstances and accomplish the goals that lie before you.

potato? Absolutely! But that's not what you are looking for, is it? You are reading this book, pledging yourself to a new way of thinking, doing, and being, and you owe it to yourself to do it right, the first time!

I always see this in the weight room: the guy or gal who is pumping out twenty to forty repetitions with bad technique. The guys (regrettably) are funnier than the ladies because they put the weight down and start to flex their muscles as they walk over to get a sip of water, full of pride with their empty accomplishment. Weeks later, I'll see the same guy doing the same workout at the same weight and unfortunately still looking the same way. No strength gains or size gains. Most people will try to make an argument against me saying that at least they can lift more than me or the next guy. Yes, that bad technique may get you a higher maximum effort, but it also gets you closer to a few other things—all of them negative.

> Picking the right routine that works for you—including exercise duration, frequency, resistance, speed, form, and schedule—is paramount for delivering results that will continue to motivate you to meet your goals.

There is such a difference between being in the gym, exercising at home, walking around the block, or hiking, and actually actively participating in your life change. Thirty minutes of aggressive, deliberate, and specific body sculpting and fat burning activity is so much more beneficial than just thirty minutes of monotonous *shucking and jiving*. You need to make valuable use of your time. Picking the right routine that works for you—including exercise duration, frequency, resistance, speed, form, and schedule—is paramount for delivering results that will continue to motivate you to meet your goals. There is nothing worse than seeing changes early on just because you have altered a few things and then leveling off (what most people call plateauing). Stay there too long, and eventually you will call it quits.

Form and technique is everything when it comes to strength training, including cardiovascular output as well. If you are the person who likes to do bicep curls halfway down and then come back up without providing the maximal lengthening of that muscle, you're shortchanging yourself big time. You could actually be doing more harm than good. There are two reasons why:

1. Muscle has both a flexibility and a strength component to it. The more flexible a muscle is, the higher the potential it has to perform better. Athletes who increase their flexibility normally have secondary increases in performance as well. Now there are some cases where stretching a muscle too much limits its ability to generate enough force to move heavier weight. That is due to a strength/flexibility relationship where tighter muscle fibers/spindles are needed for shorter, more powerful contractions. Professional weight lifters need to be more cognizant of this than the average person trying to work out in the weight room.

2. The potential for muscle injury is huge when performing exercises with improper form. Muscle performs best at or near its resting length. When a person performs a muscle contraction, the strongest part of that contraction takes places right

around the middle of the range of motion. That's because the muscle belly is taking the majority of the weight upon itself, minus the tension given off to the tendons.

As the range of motion increases or decreases, that tension is passed off to the tendons, which are intended mainly to produce adequate tension to keep the muscle from tearing. As a matter of fact, the Golgi tendon organ within that muscle belly is programmed to shut the muscle down in the presence of dangerously high levels of tension that could cause injury. Continuously flailing through repetitions and using gravity and inertia to move weight, along with shortening end ranges, make you more susceptible to dampening the response of the Golgi tendon and allowing injury to occur.

Now I know that last part may have gone over your head a bit, but trust me when I say that performing exercises with less weight and using good technique, especially when just starting an exercise plan, is paramount in generating strength gains early on.

I remember one time while I was at the University of Miami competing in track and field, the football team recruited a new strength and conditioning coach. The first thing he did was have the team log their bench press and squat maximal lifts. Then he looked at their form. The majority, if not all of them, were performing both of the exercises incorrectly. He had them strip the weight off the bar and showed them how to do it the right way. All of the maximal lift amounts plunged, but as time went by, they rose to even higher levels than before, with less muscle injuries occurring during the football season.

It carries over to cardiovascular training as well. As human beings, we move by the size principle. We recruit smaller muscles first, calling on the larger ones for help only when it is necessary to move heavier weights. Therefore, improper lifting not only puts smaller muscles at risk for injury, but it also doesn't properly allow the safe transition from small to large muscles when performing heavier lifts. This can cause larger muscle groups to be ineffectively contracted out of sync, which can add stress and cause injury.

A Closer Look

Utilizing the proper technique produces results faster. You can get stronger, work more efficiently, and melt away fat at a higher rate (sometimes in less time at the gym) if you pay close attention to proper execution. Since no one is built the same, finding the *sweet spot* for exercise conditioning can be tricky. You have to find out what works for *you*. The vital balance between working too hard and not enough has many variables, but using proper form and technique is the foundation of increasing strength and flexibility at a pace that is manageable.

There are more than six hundred plus muscles and two hundred plus bones in the human body. The muscles run from one part of a bone to another (origin and insertion), sometimes crossing one to two joints, and are responsible for different actions. The coordination between muscle groups is a fascinating phenomenon that should naturally occur. Sometimes, however, there are muscle imbalances that take place during a specific movement, with one muscle that acts (agonist), and the opposite muscle that should be in a state of relaxing (antagonist), which predisposes you to discomfort or, in some cases, injury. To battle this, I like to recommend for people to include in their exercise routine a good mix of isometric, eccentric, and concentric muscle contractions. Here are some quick descriptions of each contraction:

- *Isometric*—force production in which muscle tension occurs but without any significant displacement or movement around the joint. The muscle does not produce enough force to move the object that is resisting it.[1]

- *Concentric*—shortening of a muscle during force production, with movement noted around the joint to move the resistance.[2]

- *Eccentric*—results in the lengthening of the muscle, while the muscle simultaneously produces force in an attempt to counter the resistance imposed upon the muscle.[3]

These differing types of muscle contractions require various muscle fibers, spindles, bundles, and muscle groups to fire synchronously to produce force. Therefore performing all three types of contraction, for let's say the bicep (responsible for bending the upper arm at the elbow), allows every part of the bicep to work, decreasing the likelihood of injury, increasing strength gains, and improving flexibility.

In a study by Jerrold Petrofsky, PhD, and others, the researchers wanted to find out if co-contraction of agonist and antagonist muscle pairs while the subject is standing would be a good means of isometric strength training. In other words, is it essential to have heavy gym equipment to produce optimal results of strength training? The inference is that adding isometric muscle contractions is beneficial for producing satisfactory outcomes with strength training.

Petrofsky examined six male and eleven female subjects between the ages of twenty-two and twenty-eight, and asked them to co-contract (isometric activation of both agonist and antagonist muscles/groups) in three areas of the body (arms, trunk, and legs), and compared the results with those produced with exercises on commercial weight lifting equipment.[4] The isometric contractions were performed over three intervals of twenty-five seconds. To determine sufficient muscle activation, electromyography was utilized, providing information of muscle activity.

Overall, it was concluded that isometric exercise against agonist and antagonist pairs provides a good exercise regimen. Not only does it produce high levels of muscle tension,[5] it also allows the muscle to use glucose (sugars) and glycogen for energy versus protein,[6] increases synthesis of muscles (actin and myosin),[7] increases muscle strength,[8] and allowed for up to 15.9 times the exercise for differing muscles groups than did the commercial weight lifting.[9]

This proves that conventional exercise with commercial weight machines alone—which normally only utilizes concentric and eccentric forms of lifting—is not as beneficial as adding isometric lifts. So adding isometrics to, say, your abdominal routine is a great way to maximize sculpting that six-pack from the keg that you may be housing in the midsection.

Manuel Monfort-Panego, along with other researchers, studied the activation and synthesis of the abdominal muscles with certain exercises, collecting more than eighty-seven research articles.[10] Though most of the articles proved to be inconclusive as to what exercises are best to perform, the overall interpretation proved that efficacy of abdominal exercises increases with:

- Spine flexion and rotation without hip flexion
- Arm support
- Lower-body segments involvement controlling the correct performance
- Inclined planes or additional loads

The one big take-home point that sticks out here is the importance of technique during abdominal exercise to obtain desirable outcomes. This echoes the point I made earlier concerning the value of good technique. It cannot be underrated nor ignored. Executing exercises correctly will improve your performance and give you the results you are looking for.

Parting Gift

As my parting gift in this chapter to you as you begin to determine the correct technique and form for your exercise regimen, here are my suggestions.

The DOs of Weight Lifting and Exercise

1. Lift an appropriate amount of weight. Start with a weight you can lift comfortably twelve to fifteen times. As you get stronger, gradually increase the amount of weight.

2. Use proper form. If you're unable to maintain good form, decrease the weight or the number of repetitions.

3. Breathe. Holding your breath can lead to dangerous increases in blood pressure. Instead, breathe out as you lift the weight, and breathe in as you lower the weight.

4. Seek balance. Work all of your major muscles—abdominals, legs, chest, back, shoulders, and arms.

5. Rest. Avoid exercising the same muscles two days in a row.

I know, I know. I can hear you from here (at home, in front of my computer as you read this book wherever you are—which is weird because we've never met and I wrote this way before you ever thought about getting this book). I'm babbling. Sorry. Let's get to the point. You're saying this sounds simple on paper, but what about reality? Everything sounds easy until you try it. Ever hear about that guy who walked on water? Or the one who split the Red Sea? Sure, those sound simple when you read them, but the application is a beast. I know this, so I added a few additional tips to get you started. Beware, another acronym is approaching.

- **A**: Ask for help. It may take a few sessions with a certified personal trainer to get you started in the right direction. Learning *how* to exercise effectively makes all the difference.

- **C**: Capture the powerful moments and make good on them. Not all days are going to be amazing. Some days you just won't feel like working out.

But on the good ones, when you feel energized and pumped, take advantage of it. Work out like an animal. Do two or three extra sets if you feel like it. This way, when you have a bad day, you won't feel as bad about giving half the effort. There is nothing wrong with making fitness deposits on your health.

- **E:** Expense management is paramount. Once you start cutting back on eating the wrong things, make a commitment to spend money on what is going to make you healthier. Food, gym memberships, and workout equipment are neither free nor cheap. Slowly work everything into your budget that makes sense. Prioritize your health first over your junk. You can stand to pass on buying things for pleasure for a few months to focus on getting better. Later on in the book, you'll read about my campaign that will help you save money while getting in shape.

Chapter 12

BROKEN CLOCK

I OFTEN GET FRUSTRATED when I hear people quote parables and sayings, especially the ones that are supposed to encourage you. Most times it just seems like someone is trying to mock you or make light of your struggles. My favorite terrible one is: "It's always darkest before the dawn." Wow, that's deep. Is that really supposed to help others pull themselves out of the jaws of despair if they are feeling low? Is that truly something that will enable that person to collect himself or herself and be inspired to look past failures and patiently await eventual success? I guess we are waiting for that person to say, "Well, I was wondering why things were so grim and dreary. I guess I can sit back and relax and wait for the lights to come on soon."

What do we offer them in the meantime? No one can ever be a victor if they continue to walk in mediocrity and just do nothing. Offering someone rudimentary words of advice that have been handed down century after century, without giving them an ounce of advice about what to do, is as good as giving a drowning man a picture of oxygen—comforting but not acceptable. We have to give them more than that. Much less, we need to give ourselves more than that as well.

We need words of encouragement that are action based. Merely speaking to someone else about how things will be better someday or even encouraging yourself with empty analogies is not profitable. We have to have plans for the future—plans that outline our path to glory.

Now the only problem with having plans, even of God's design, is that this tiny little element called *time* exists. If things seem as if they are moving slowly, too slowly for you, fret not. God controls time, and contrary to what you may be thinking, the clock is not broken. It is only moving at the speed that is most fitting. It's just too bad for us that the speed of something happening doesn't fall within the lines of our expectancy.

I want to implant an action word in your mind that will sustain you when times get tough. It will get you off the couch, and galvanize you to act. No longer will you be a pincushion to the jaggy exploits of life. You will know how to exist in the moment, live for the now, conquer your fears, and defeat that which seeks to destroy you. The word is *love*.

> God controls time, and contrary to what you may be thinking, the clock is not broken.

Empower Your Mind With Love

You need to learn how to love yourself. Love works in sync with time. Time is good because it is the essence of development. We learn skills through our experiences, grow into maturity, and persevere through our struggles. It only happens with time. But a byproduct of time is love. Love takes time to cultivate. Like a beautiful flower that sprouts in the spring and blossoms in the summer, love starts off small. As it continues to be nurtured and cared for it springs forth roots that dig deeper into the soil. The petals expand, widening with the expectation of hope. As it reaches forth toward the sky, the stem strengthens, making that flower sturdier so it can withstand the blows of uncertainty.

I want to challenge you to love three things, more than you ever knew you had the capacity to love.

1. Love yourself.

This isn't about being conceited, arrogant, or pompous. It's about respecting the person that you have become over time. Time worked hard at making you who you are today. It took seconds, minutes, days, weeks, months, and years of planning. Looking at who you are today gives you a baseline, something to work with. I know that a lot of you who are reading this part right here have been through some terrible times. Some of the things are so painful that it is a daily fight for you to drown out the mental imagery that still haunts you today. But while those struggles may have weakened you, *they couldn't break you*. Somehow, someway, you maintained and made it through the storm. The summation of events that shaped you gave you the tools that you can now use to embrace your success.

The next step is to clean the slate. Wipe away all the emotional scars that have stunted your growth. If you are a person who is in a relationship and feels that you cannot let another person get close to you because someone else hurt you before, let that go. You can change the way you think. We all enter this world with our minds on a clean tablet, waiting for the programs to be downloaded so that we can modulate to the inner workings of our own psyche. So just because you are comfortable because you don't like to openly love someone else doesn't mean that you cannot. You are just protecting yourself, and it's time to love yourself enough to let someone love you more. You'll never let them do that if you do not love yourself *first*.

2. Love others.

Love even those who hurt you. Keeping those feelings of resentment built up inside of you just takes up space. You could easily use that room to store up things like love, peace, and joy. Hating or disliking others slows your development, allowing time to weigh you down. Have you ever felt like the days just drag on, moving at a snail's pace? If you do, think about the condition of your heart. Are there people who have a hold on you emotionally? When you see them or even hear someone talk about them, does the lining inside your stomach twist up, making you want to ball up your fist and take a swing at something? That emotion is so heavy that it adds to the weight of the day. It's like walking a marathon with a spare five-pound weight strapped to your back. It doesn't slow you down so much in the beginning, but after a while, you start to experience the effects.

Love them; let the pain, anger, and fear go. Then your days will begin to fly by. You'll start to see life in a new light, and begin to desire longer days.

3. Love the time.

Appreciate the moments. Time can either steal from you or give to you. When you are running late for work, time doesn't seem to help. Minutes sail by like seconds, making you feel encumbered with anxiety. When you are enjoying life, time steals the instances from you, shortening the sweetness. But learn to love time itself. Time in the gym, time at work, time with loved ones (even the ones that get on your nerves). Time is profitable for learning, teaching, refining, molding, shaping, and building those things that are necessary for you to grow into the person you need to be to realize your purpose. Even appreciate getting older. Hopefully with time came wisdom, so you know exactly where I'm coming from.

So what happens when the clock seems to be broken? A moment when time stands still and the opportunities of success are nowhere to be found. Nothing new is growing, everything appears to be dying, and life itself will not give you a break. Stop looking at the clock and begin to focus on your efforts. Prioritize the moments, and make the most of them. Act as if you have no time. Live as though you are on borrowed time. That way

> Time is profitable for learning, teaching, refining, molding, shaping, and building those things that are necessary for you to grow into the person you need to be to realize your purpose.

you will have nothing to offer but your utmost best, valuing every drop of sweat and degree of energy you exert for every task. That way, you can be assured that what comes to fruition will only be the best because it came out of your best. Be proud of the product that you are. You are a product of time itself.

COSBY'S CORNER
Processed Before the Procession

Boy, here's one for the ages. People nowadays are heading for the funeral home at a rate alarmingly disturbing, rivaling that of the rate of folks going to the doctor for an annual checkup. Answer this question: Why is it that people need warning shots or a wake-up call before they start to take their health seriously?

I mean, really, people, does it take the midnight phone call from the police telling you that your son or daughter has been pulled over to the side of the road and is under arrest for driving under the influence to make us notice that they are crying out for help? Or do we have to make a trip to the hospital to visit Grandpa who just underwent a triple bypass surgery to get the courage to tell him that he needs to watch his diet?

I know the old saying goes, "It is always darkest before the dawn," but we shouldn't use that as the lighthouse on the island sanctuary while we navigate the treacherous waters of our daily lives. Nobody should be wearing this ideal as a bumper sticker on the back of the car, or tattooed across the chest like it is some type of colloquialism. We need to wake up! We are all desensitizing ourselves to the stark reality that our behaviors, diets, habits, and lifestyles are slowly killing us. We are being processed before the procession.

I like to think for a moment about the self-made diabetic folks out there. Not all of them, just the people who have feasted on high-calorie diets, blindly cruising along until their doctor diagnoses them one day with type 2 diabetes. Who do we blame? Is it entirely their fault, or is it something more insidious lying beneath the surface of the truth? Should these folks be allowed to write a letter to the fast food industry or the food processing plants and ask for their money back?

I mean, let's keep it real here for a minute. I am not saying that they are innocent, because they did make the decision to eat the stuff, but it's not like a majority of people or businesses are trying to change the status quo of what is going on in America. There are very few who are doing so, and they lack support from the majority.

You get diagnosed, you realize you have to make life changes, monitor your blood sugar daily (which requires sticking yourself with a needle), and these billion-dollar corporations got rich at your expense. And they didn't even have the nerve to send you a thank you note. Process before the procession!

Don't forget the holidays! Thanksgiving, Christmas, New Years, and Fourth of July are all excuses for people to stuff their faces in celebration. Celebration of what?

I'm sorry, but please do not have anyone scarf down multiple layers of saturated fats and artery-clogging volleys of cholesterol and say they are doing it on my behalf. I'd be just as happy with them eating a bowl of broccoli or a cup of yogurt. Don't do me any favors.

On a serious note, have you seen what people bring to these occasions? It's like there is a secret contest or hidden game show going on between the cooks of the family: Let's Make a Processed Deal or The Slice Is Right are two that come to mind. You don't believe me? Check out what is left on the table after everyone has finished eating. The spinach salad, broccoli casserole, and string beans are somewhere between half to full in their respective bowls. While the macaroni and cheese, fried chicken, and sweet potato pies (you know they didn't use fresh sweet potatoes) are nowhere to be found. Now here is the real moment of sadness: everyone is too tired to clean up after the meal. Most are slumped over on the couch catching a few zzzz's. And they have the nerve to blame the poor turkey for it. No, that's not it at all. It's because your body has shunted the majority of blood away from your brain to your digestive system in an attempt to break down all that processed stuff you just shoveled into it.

Now let's take a bigger step forward and talk about the theme parks. Vending machines, fried cookies (c'mon man), candy apples, funnel cake, cotton candy, chicken fingers, and carbonated beverages and slushies all make for a marvelous selection of foods, which slaps an exclamation point for a beautiful time with family and friends. Yet all the while, you've probably pumped yourself with more than five thousand calories of eye and mouth pleasure and nothing beneficial to the body. And guess what, the kids want to come back tomorrow. Why wouldn't they? They just got juiced up on enough sugary voltage to run a small wonderland power plant. Can't blame them now, can we? But I can blame you for letting this madness play out.

Now I know what you are going to say, "It's not like we take them every day, and they are just kids." I definitely side with you on this, but here is the mistake: we view the negative as something acceptable just because we've been conditioned to accept it. It's not like we have activists standing outside of the theme parks, fast food restaurants, and the food processing plants with picket signs screaming, "Repent, for the end is nigh." We save those types of tasks for the "tree hugger society" and "save the whales" groups.

The truth is that genocide is happening every day right in our own backyards (barbecue grills included). So, I am going to make a stand right now and beckon that you rise from your slumber and decide to rage against the machine. Walk with me down the path that leads to good health, long life, and peace of mind, so that you, your children, and your children's children can break this cycle of being processed before the procession. If anything, let's all make the undertaker's job a little bit harder. I'm just saying . . .

■■■

Go to Your Spirit's Source

With most of our day-to-day hectic scheduling, we often find ourselves in a mad dash to get everything done and never seem to accomplish anything we set out to do. Our plates are way too full, we are too busy, and we lack the structural organization it takes to systematically meet the requirements of each task. Our task analysis breaks down somewhere, and we are unable to tell if our performance is what it should be or should've been to produce fair gains. If that sounds like a business performance portfolio to you, you're right. Most people handle all of their acts of daily living like a business. The line between work and life becomes blurred, making it impossible to operate one without the other. But this can be beneficial if you know where to exert your energies in the right place and in the correct capacity. You need a source of focus outside of your constant juggling and labor to bring it all together. That source is and has to be God.

God tells us about prioritizing throughout the Bible. The sickness of being a busy body can be distracting, taking the focus off of the Giver and only on the gifts. We get so entangled in our own web of desires to have more that we neglect the source of where it all comes from. But I especially like what Jesus prescribes for us to follow in Matthew 6:33–34, "But seek first the kingdom of God and His righteousness, and all these things shall be given to you. Therefore, take no thought about tomorrow, for tomorrow will take thought about the things of itself. Sufficient to the day is the trouble thereof."

Jesus instructs us to seek the kingdom of God first. This has to be the center of our efforts. Getting into a strong relationship with God allows His perfect will to work in us and through us. Our destination cannot be more important than our point of origin. Even though we may want to ponder on the causes and effects of the system, what is truly the most valuable piece is the starting point. Is your foundation stable? Do you have your feet planted firmly in truth? Are you so worried about outcomes and the objective of satisfying your own pride that you've gotten away from the vision that God may have already given you?

God wants to bless us, all of us. But most times we struggle to make God line up with what we feel should happen next and how it should happen. As long as we keep seeking God, He is delighted to show us everything. He has the keys to the kingdom and time itself. He can speed things up, or He can bring them

> Getting into a strong relationship with God allows His perfect will to work in us and through us.

to a snail's pace if He has to. He doesn't do this as punishment but sometimes He does it to teach and save us from ourselves and happenstance.

Sometimes I have to thank God for delaying things because, looking back, if He had given me everything at once I would have seriously messed it up. My ignorance of the matter would have sent things in the opposite direction, tainting God's plan entirely. But thank God that He is faithful. In our weak efforts, He is strong. As we reach forth to take a prize of the earthly, natural things, He pulls them back and gives more spiritual blessing, so that we can be satisfied with that which is more essential for the time being. That way, when we finally receive the natural things, we are able to handle and appreciate it more. Then we can be giving and honor God with our firstfruits.

Jesus also warns that we should not be anxious over time. Man, oh, man. I know that He was talking about me in verse 34. I get so anxious about the time windows, wondering when things are going to happen. I don't doubt that God can do all that He says He will do; I just wonder when He is going to tell me to do my part. As time crawls by, I start to think to myself that He must be waiting on me to do something. It becomes so hard to just sit and wait and allow for His power to flow. God can raise up rocks and donkeys to do His bidding. How much less does He need us to chip in and *help Him* out? Our reliance on God to do what He has promised in the Bible and spoken to us through dreams and visions and even others, is paramount. It demonstrates our level of trust in Him as our Father and Savior. We can surely diminish that trust by jumping in and getting our hands dirty. God, being a gracious Father, just steps back and lets us do all our little efforts. Sometimes, I can hear Him in the background saying, "Go ahead, Braxton, keep on doing it. When you are done and ready to let Me do My thing, I will."

How do we stay focused, even when we are beginning to build this relationship and seek His kingdom? We dwell on His laws. His ways are perfect, and His laws are divine. He pleads that we should always make it our practice to follow what He has entrusted the men of old to create in the Bible. In Proverbs 3:1–6 God says:

> My son, do not forget my teaching,
>> but let your heart keep my commandments;
> for length of days and long life
>> and peace will they add to you.
>
> Do not let mercy and truth forsake you;
>> bind them around your neck,
>> write them on the tablet of your heart,
> so you will find favor and good understanding
>> in the sight of God and man.
>
> Trust in the LORD with all your heart,
>> and lean not on your own understanding;
> in all your ways acknowledge Him,
>> and He will direct your paths.

First of all, God confirms our relation to Him as child by calling us sons. Then He tells us not to forget His laws and to keep His commandments. There would be no way to play the game properly without knowing the rules. Therefore, how can we live in expectation of the promises of God without first knowing the laws that God governs the world, universe, and heavens with? God has set forth a perfect system with provision available to those who earnestly seek Him (Matt. 6:33), and those who write that system upon their hearts can receive favor and good understanding. With those things being established, God asks us to trust Him with everything we have, especially our hearts.

Remember earlier in the chapter when I asked you to love others and most of all yourself? There is a level of trust that has to be given, not with man but with God. If we trust Him to be everything to us, then we can forgive others and love people without the fear of them hurting us, because essentially, we are doing what God has called us to do in His command- ments: love others as we love ourselves. God cannot divide Himself. He is the living Word. He cannot first tell us to do something and then allow that same commandment to bring us harm. It would cause His words to collapse.

I love to use a passage of Scripture from the Book of Habakkuk as inspiration when I'm trying to wait on God to bring a vision to fruition. In Habakkuk 2:2–3, God specifically answers the prophet Habakkuk concerning a request he made of the Lord. God says, "Write the vision, and make it plain on tablets, that he who reads it may run. For the vision is yet for an appointed time; but it speaks of the end, and does not lie. If it delays, wait for it; it will surely come, it will not delay."

God's promises, visions, and revelations are absolute. He exists outside of the realm of time, so He knows the appointed time of when it will come to pass.

We mess it up when we lose hope and stop believing. We walk away and forget the vision. This is why He commanded Habakkuk to write it down on tablets. Tablets back in biblical days were forged from stone and marble. Our tablets today are made of fancy circuitry and technology and can be deleted at any time. But God is speaking to us today at a level more figurative than literal. The *tablet* spiritually represents fortifying the Word and declaration of God on something permanent. Make it real and plain. Hold on to the promise that your healing is coming; your breakthrough is near; your family is healed; your body, soul, and mind are complete; and your season of reaping is at hand. He declares that at the appointed time it will certainly not delay. But—and there is always a *but*—there is a stipulation. Verse 1 of the same chapter defines this: "I will stand at my watch and station myself on the watchtower; and I will keep watch to see what He will say to me."

Habakkuk knew that he had to make the first move. There was a requirement that he take his position, his watch, his assigned post, and see what God would tell him. You have to do the same. Make yourself available to hear from God, to receive the healing, and to prosper in time of lack. Then and only then will you be able to have what is promised.

Finally God requires that we acknowledge Him in all that we do. That way we can assure that He will direct our paths. Losing weight? Acknowledge Him as your strength. Improving your glucose and cholesterol levels? Acknowledge Him for healing. Are your finances improving? Acknowledge Him as a provider. Relationship mending? Acknowledge Him as the source of resolution. Then, He will be able to guide you in the direction you need to follow for even more victory beyond even what you imagined.

Working everything out takes time. And we must wait patiently for the results because we know that everything is in His hands, and He is just to reward us for our diligence. Keeping our goals in front of us, maintaining our focus on

God, and trusting in His provision for our lives will direct our paths, and we shall reap our just rewards.

The Importance of Time to Your Body

The main focus of this chapter thus far has centered on time and the value of utilizing each precious moment to get the most out of life. Whether working out in the gym, completing a task for work, or even being with your loved ones, we have to make a decision to be the best that we possibly can within the measurable component of time. So let's take a closer look at the importance of applying that measure as it pertains to weight loss.

> Losing weight? Acknowledge Him as your strength. Improving your glucose and cholesterol levels? Acknowledge Him for healing. Are your finances improving? Acknowledge Him as a provider.

Most experts collectively agree that the only way to assure that weight stays off is by making life changes that center on food, lifestyle, and habits. It may hurt a little in the beginning, but like most things that are taken away from us, we learn to adapt. That's what separates human beings from any other animal on the planet. We are able to adapt to situations, assess the probability for success, and then make the necessary changes to put the odds in our favor.

I know that you may have tried all of these crazy diets and food substitutes in hopes that it will make you shed pounds as easily as a snake sheds its skin, but alas, I'm sure you realized that those techniques only made you even more frustrated. If you have tried the slow and steady approach, how did it go for you? Have you taken the time to step back from the situation and ascertain the pitfalls that caused you to lose out? There are many factors that probably set you back—workout scheduling, meal planning, and volume control. Even though these are critical for making a realistic life change, the most important piece of the puzzle is you. Did you really commit to all the fine details that would have set you up for success? Or did you focus on just one or two and hope that your efforts would somehow make up for your lack of dedication?

When it comes to weight loss, you cannot cut corners. There is no lightning in a bottle method that can substitute for good old-fashioned hard work—other than, say, surgery, which not everyone can afford. And with surgery, there are lifestyle modifications required to ensure that the surgery yields the best results.

> When it comes to weight loss, you cannot cut corners. There is no lightning in a bottle method that can substitute for good old-fashioned hard work.

The story of the tortoise and the hare is the best illustration of putting this into practice. Look at it this way: it took years to put the weight on so it's going to take the same if not more time to burn it off.

We already know the benefits of exercise, and I've touched on the importance of volume control in the earlier chapter. But we also need to consider the content of the food we consume as a powerful component of maintaining the weight loss. You do not want to be a statistic and become a victim of the *yo-yo* effect of dieting—losing a lot of weight and then putting it all back on, if not even more, over time. The only way to predict successful long-term maintenance of weight loss is by closely monitoring all three components.

In a study by Rena R. Wing and James O. Hill, they looked closely at obese subjects who lost weight and the trends that were associated with long-term weight loss. First, they consider successful long-term weight loss as anyone losing at least 10 percent of their initial body weight and keeping it off for more than one year.[1] They combed through the National Weight Control Registry (NWCR)—a registry of three thousand individuals who have been extremely successful at long-term weight loss maintenance—to disseminate the correlating positive factors for obtaining weight loss maintenance.

To be eligible for the NWCR, you must have maintained at least a thirty-pound weight loss for at least one year. The participants were asked to complete several questionnaires in an effort to understand maintenance behaviors, as well as history, quality of life, and demographic information.[2]

> Most people who lose weight seem to do so on their own, without participation in any formalized programs.

Overall there seems to be a feeling of pessimism regarding long-term weight loss.[3] A sample of one hundred obese individuals were referred to a nutritional weight loss program and, after two years, only 2 percent of the participants kept off at least twenty pounds.[4]

Pessimism aside, there is potential to keep the weight off, especially if you get serious about it and take the accountability and place the responsibility in your hands. Most people who lose weight seem to do so on their own, without participation in any formalized programs.[5]

After collecting the data, Wing and Hill discovered that there was a distinct similarity in the strategies imposed to successfully lose weight:

• Eating a diet low in fat

• Regular physical activity

• Frequent self-monitoring

It is no surprise that consuming a low-fat diet and increasing the amount of regular activity helped maintain weight loss, but let's concentrate on the third component: self-monitoring.[6] Registry members frequently monitored their weight. Some reported doing so daily (44 percent) and some did so weekly (31 percent). As a matter of fact, weight loss is consistent with self-monitoring.[7]

> The scale has to become your best friend. You have to face it every week and determine that it is going to reflect the hard work you have put in.

I do not recommend daily weighing in early on because it seems to have a discouraging effect on people I work with. I suggest at least once a week, at the same time, wearing the same clothing, and using the same scale. But the study makes the correlation between people who have already successfully lost the weight and are keeping it off by keeping a close eye on their weight. The last thing you need is to meet your goals, slack off a little, and then run from the scale. The scale has to become your best friend. You have to face it every week and determine that it is going to reflect the hard work you have put in.

The consensus is very clear: the only way to maintain weight loss is to develop routines that are habit forming. Addressing the three strategies listed above, *over time*, is paramount in allowing you to not just lose weight but also keep it off. Crash diets are just that, crashing, and fad diets fade. Not only that, but the data suggests that fluctuating weight up and down over many years can put you at an even greater risk for coronary heart disease. Carefully select a plan that works for you, and make preparations to stick with it. Don't let all your hard work go down the drain. You deserve better and owe it to yourself to be better. Yo-yos just aren't that fun anyway.

Chapter 13

REALIZE YOUR STRENGTH

HAVE YOU EVER been up against an opponent you were fully convinced you could not defeat? I mean, really, think about it for a second. You are there, back against the wall, time running out, filled with nothing but despair and unabated loss staring you smack in the face. What happened? What did you do about it? Was it truly the end? Did you somehow overcome it? Maybe you won; maybe you lost. But somewhere, somehow, in the end, you actually made it through to see another day. You want to know how I know? Because you are here reading this book today.

Yeah, I know it's kind of a cheap trick. The only way I'm assured that you survived is because you lived to tell the tale—or at least to read this excerpt. The truth is, many of us project that things will be worse than they are, and in the end, it usually falls short of the condemning thoughts of our minds. But that is where the power really lies: in our thoughts.

Develop the Power of a Positive Mind

You are what you believe yourself to be. Looking at every situation as an opportunity to first learn, then receive something from the experience whether good or bad, allows us to grow. We are enabled to grow in faith, grow in wisdom, and grow in maturity. These things pour the foundation of our being. As the growth takes place, the strength that you already possess inside of you begins to pour out. It spills over onto other people. They become infected with the outbreak of positive energy, and you become saturated in the power of inspiration and encouragement. Your personal testimony becomes the basis for someone else's growth.

Anyone can read Bible verses, preach a ready-made sermon, or even spout off inspirational quotes all day. If those words do not penetrate into the heart of the person hearing it, they are merely words on a paper—symbols without substance. The person hears you, politely allows you to finish, and walks away unchanged. What makes the difference is your conviction. You have to become passionate in your calling. Believe beyond what you can *see* with your eyes, and rely only on what you *feel* in your heart. Your strength stems from your faith.

I am just starting to understand how this faith thing really works. It can't just be based on God, or on yourself. There has to be a mixing of the two. How can someone believe in the majestic glory of God and hold fast to His promises to be blessed without first trusting in them? If an individual only relies on his or her own judgments and abilities and denies the power of God, making his or her existence only about self, what room have they allowed for the promises and glory of

God? The one cannot live without the other. You must equally believe in both yourself and God.

Believe in:

- *Yourself*—to appreciate the power that God has bestowed in you to do something significant for His purpose

- *God*—to fully receive the individual calling that He has placed in your life to do something magnificent. How can you believe what God is going to do in the spiritual if you lack the confidence to carry it out in the natural?

The two ideals will be in opposition of one another and will ultimately clash, sending the framework of faith crashing to the floor. We must believe beyond what we see with our eyes today, and what we experienced in the past, and step into the vision of the future—the tomorrows—that God has in store for us, which will unlock our faith, which is our strength.

I remember the first race I ever ran my freshman year in college at the University of Miami. We were competing at the University of Florida. I was frightened almost unto death. My body shook with fear—of what, I do not fully know. All I did know was

> We must believe beyond what we see with our eyes today

that my stomach never settled inside my gut, making me feel like I had eaten a bowl of lively goldfish.

I warmed up, two, three, four times as much as I needed to. I did anything I could to shake the nervousness away. But it never left me. Finally, they called my heat in the 55-meter hurdles, and it seemed as if someone pulled the power cord to the sound system of the world. I went deaf. My hands poured sweat, and I immediately ran to the starting blocks and set my measurements. I didn't even look at the other competitors. I couldn't! A couple of quick starts, and my body began to ease a little. I was doing what made me feel comfortable.

I took off my warm ups and stripped down to my uniform. The shaking stopped—finally. Taking one last deep breath, I looked around at the other runners in their lanes, and it happened. The shaking returned. Right next to me was what I believed to the biggest human being on the planet. Everything about him was big. Arms, legs, shoes, and even his numbers seemed to stand out in 3-D. His uniform barely fit, stretching to the point of transparency. All I could ask myself was, "Why is he in the lane next to me?"

> Setting the hope of desirable outcomes low predetermines the results. You handcuff both God and yourself when you do that.

I automatically knew I was racing for second place. What do you think happened? I'll release you from the suspense and tell you. I beat him. I didn't win the race, but I did beat him. As a matter of fact, I think I hit every hurdle in front of him. The lesson here is about my expectations. I allowed myself to be intimidated by the flesh. His size mattered to me. Nothing about *me* made a difference. I discounted my own strength and power because of what he looked like.

Setting the hope of desirable outcomes low predetermines the results. You handcuff both God and yourself when you do that. Going into any fight with one arm strapped behind your back never makes for a competitive slugfest. It only creates an atmosphere of failure. Realize your strength and walk in it. I can't define where that exactly is, but one thing I am certain of is this: it lies somewhere in the destination between you and God. And faith is the key to unlocking your internal navigation system, which will give you the turn-by-turn directions to finding it. My uncle has a great quote to summarize this: "Decide that you want it more than you are afraid of it." I concur.

COSBY'S CORNER
The Fear of Mr. T

Have you ever had a real fear? I mean, it didn't matter how much you convinced yourself that it wasn't real, your fear always came back to kick you dead in the face and say, "Here I am!" You couldn't ignore it. It haunted your mind like an angry yellow jacket trying to protect its nest, stinging at your thoughts.

I have had that fear more than once in my life, but one that is particularly terrifying to me involved a modern-day superhero. That's right, Mr. T, folks. Yeah, I know, it doesn't make any sense. If you are reading this and are of the age of thirty or higher, you know who the celebrity is. He was made very famous from the old action TV show *The A-Team*. As much as he was a huge, menacing personality, he has a real sweet side to him. I used to even watch his cartoon show that he had with some gymnasts that solved crimes. I was a fan. I didn't fear Mr. T, the man. I feared his head.

Let me explain. I used to be a part of the Boy Scouts while growing up. Even though my troop did little to nothing, we always seemed to raise a few funds to throw a Christmas party. This was going to be a great time: friends, family, food, and, of course, gifts. The gift exchange would be in the form of a grab bag. You buy your toy, place it in the bag, and at the end of the party, everyone would come forward, reach in a bag, and pull out a gift. It was an easy venture. No muss, no fuss, right? Wrong!

My mother bought a cool toy, some kind of G. I. Joe action figure, with extra Kung-Fu grip, cool weapons, and articulated elbows and forearms so that he could shoot his gun at multiple angles. I recall thinking that everyone was going to buy a gift this cool. That way, we all could have some neat takeaway from the party. We were Boy Scouts, for crying out loud. We would look out for our fellow scouts and hook them up with something cool, right? Wrong!

As the party winds down, the troop leader begins to collect the toys and place them in the larger-than-life garbage bag. A friend of mine leaned over and whispered in my ear, "Hey, look, somebody brought a Mr. T piggy bank as a gift. I hope I don't get that one." It was hideous. If Mr. T knew that thing existed, he would have surely had Hannibal make some ingenious plan to destroy the manufacturing plant behind it so that no kid would ever have to endure using it—ever. The rest of the troop saw it as well, erupting into muffled snickers and giggles. I responded, "Man, I feel sorry for the poor kid who pulls that thing out" (foreshadowing here, folks).

It was showtime. One by one, scout after scout, we lined up and pressed forward, inching closer and closer to the bag. Ten scouts down, and no one pulled that monstrosity of a head out of the bag yet. Five more scouts went by and the head was nowhere to be found. How deep was that garbage bag anyway? My friend leaned over my shoulder and offered some advice, "Feel around in the bag first, and then pull out the smallest toy you can." I slowly nodded my head in agreement. That's when the troop leader made an announcement.

"Guys, this is taking too long. We don't have time for you to feel around in the bag. Just reach your hand inside, pull out a toy, and keep it moving."

One more scout remained in front of me, and I could feel the back of my throat drying up. I took a large dry swallow and stepped forward. My head began to throb, my heart raced, and my breath quickened. I could have sworn I was about to have an asthma attack. My fear had overcome me. What if I pulled out the Mr. T head? I'd be the laughing stock of the party. Actually, I'd be that night's entertainment. It would be the one memorable topic that everyone would talk about the next day at school. I was sure that it would even trickle over into the next year's party. I could hear them later, "Hey, man, I remember when Braxton pulled out that Mr. T head. That was the funniest thing ever!" "Yeah, I wonder if he's going to pull out the rest of the A-Team this year."

I wanted to turn back and run the other way. But how could I? Everyone was watching, waiting for Mr. T to show his ugly mug. I stood dazed, paralyzed, consumed. "Reach in there, Cosby, we ain't got all night," the troop leader yelled. I slid my hand into the bag and waved it around slowly, searching the air with my fingertips. Anything small would do the trick. I distinctly remember the head calling out to me in Mr. T. fashion like one of those lines in the show, "I pity the fool who doesn't grab me. I pity him!" My hands shook.

"Now, Cosby!" the troop leader yelled again. This time, I moved, stabbing into the darkness and pulling out . . . wait for it . . . a little longer . . . the Mr. T head. The crowd exploded in laughter. My eyes filled with tears. I had nothing left in me to do but run to the arms of my mother and bury my face in her chest.

Long story short, it stunk that I was the one to take Mr. T home that night. After a while, the tragic event faded from my mind, and you know what, that Mr. T piggy bank actually turned out to be a pretty nice money collector. And no one even talked about that head ever again, except for my ex-friend—whose name I can't remember and don't wish to now.

That life lesson taught me something: whatever fears you have, it never really proves to be as bad as you project or expect it to be. You don't have to be consumed by it or by the outcomes. If you are afraid to take the necessary steps to good health, you are living out my Mr. T head experience and you need to do like I did: reach in the bag, stab into the darkness, and take a swipe at chance. It's the only way you'll ever move past your fear. Who knows, you just may end up liking the outcome just as much as I did. If you refuse to face your fear and run away, you'll only be as pathetic as a Boy Scout who leaves a Christmas party empty handed. Bank on that! I'm just saying . . .

■ ■ ■

Develop Spiritual Precision

The biblical scripture that best epitomizes the ideal of finding your strength is one that is near and dear to my heart. It was one that Grandmother always quoted to me. Whenever a big test was looming or a sporting contest was on the horizon, it would roll from her tongue, resonate in my ears, and stab into my heart with what I call *spiritual precision*. She believed in the words even if I didn't. But that didn't stop her from saying it, reciting it to me over and over again. Philippians 4:13 says, "I can do all things because of Christ who strengthens me." The repetitive words of a humble woman still echo in my mind today. What sanctuary I find them to be...to know that all things can be accomplished through the power of a risen Savior.

As to not underplay the verse by any means, I'd like to take portions of it and elaborate a bit, allowing you to fully comprehend the power of the words.

I can...

It's less scripture and more positive reinforcement. There is something about declaring something and including yourself in the message that creates a connection between dream and reality. In the text, the word *can* is used as a verbal auxiliary word. It means, "to know how to." Therefore, you can substitute and say, "I know how to," and connect it with the rest of the verse. That's an exhilarating phenomenon to consider because it means that you already have the power to do it, because it's based on experience.

How can you say you know how to do something if you never did it before? You must have some reference point. If you don't have a reference point in the natural world, then the comprehension must somehow cross over into the spiritual world.

Your spirit is very exacting, running parallel to the inference of the scripture, and confirming the inevitable truth— you can because the knowledge and strength have been given to you already. It has been predetermined, ordained, fashioned from the spoken Word at the same instance as the creation of the world itself. I encourage you to look in the mirror when you say this verse, putting special emphasis on this part.

Do all things...

Those verses don't say just some things or most things, but *all things.* Let me paint the picture for you here. It's like the first time that my wife and I went to an all-inclusive resort. We went to dinner, rented canoes, called for room service, and ate and drank just about anything we wanted whenever we wanted to. I kept waiting for someone to come around the corner and tell us that we've reached some limit or say that something was off limits. But they never did. It was truly all inclusive.

That's how this passage of Scripture is. "All things" means all things. No gimmicks, no jokes, no limits. God intends for us to grasp the concept, meditate on it, and digest it the best way we can. But it is easier said than done.

Our mortal thoughts are run by limitations. Our souls are trapped inside a fleshly body that constantly reminds us that we are fragile, weak, and at the mercy of a little thing on planet Earth called *gravity.* The definition of man is based on limitations. But what if we were to be persuaded that limitations have been revoked—that this verse is the secret to powering down gravity? We could fly, soar, and even escape the atmosphere and float into space. Could you actually believe enough to try it? What do you have to lose?

Through Christ who strengthens me

Aha! There *is* a clause. Only through Christ do we have this power. Christ is the key, our point of contact. He is the spiritual voltage that charges us. We are allowed to walk in the authority of a royal priesthood, lacking nothing and wanting for nothing. Our strength is allowed to flow out, full blast, and unabatedly. With Him we have our being. We are set free to roam and possess all the things that He has laid before us: victory, prosperity, and peace.

No other verse in the Bible personifies the magnificent reflection of God's promise to us as His children. We can rest knowing that He has already given us the strength. We have received the award ahead of time, without even having to lift a finger because it was established before time itself. It was a moment where the words *failure, loss, doubt, rejection,* and *hurt* didn't exist yet. We can get back to a time like that by merely releasing the strength in us by believing what God can and already has done for us. Taking hold of the garment of Christ to ensure your victory both in the spirit and the natural is the starting point.

We are called to be so much more than what we are, but we fail to do greater things because we believe so little. In order to fully appreciate what we are called to do, we must build our relationship with Him through faith.

> We have to accept that we are made for larger things.

Your Strength Is Not Only in Your Body

The title of this chapter emphasizes the importance of realizing your own strength, and so far, hopefully you fully comprehend that it extends beyond just the physical world. There is value in understanding the strength that dwells within you that testifies to the power that comes from inside of us all. We have to accept that we are made for larger things. There is no room for mediocrity or being *ordinary*.

Being in a place of greatness is not meant for only celebrities or role models. That plane of existence is a position that can be obtained by everyone because it only requires that you see the purpose of your life and that you have the faith and courage to walk in that calling. But when it comes to addressing the physical, you must also realize your strength because it is the only way to improve your performance. Establishing a baseline concerning your fitness is the foundation that you build upon each week, day in and day out.

> No matter what you do—changing what you eat, how much you eat, or when you eat—you will fall short of your fitness goals if you do not add strength training.

There is no point in heading to the gym every day without an understanding of how much you can lift, because it strips you of the ability to push yourself. Each bout of exercise needs to be an opportunity to climb the ladder of growth and development. Creating milestones for weight loss, strength, body composition, and BMI are invaluable measures for inspiration. You need to have a plan going in and coming out. Without it, you will continue to aimlessly work, void of direction or objectives, both of which will guarantee imminent failure and discouragement.

I've given you quite a bit to chew on in this book to whet your appetite, but I must emphasize one last piece of advice that correlates with this chapter. No matter what you do—changing what you eat, how much you eat, or when you eat—you will fall short of your fitness goals if you do not add strength training.

I know some people do not like working out to begin with,

and it's a chore to even get you to do some light walking around the neighborhood, so if that is you, you must be asking the question, "How does he expect me to lift weights if I barely like walking or jogging?" The answer to the question is simple. Strength training is the hidden gem that everyone who has successfully lost weight and kept it off is doing. It's true! The principles behind it are intricate, but simple at the same time. Let me explain it to you as simply as I can.

Lean muscle mass is built up based on the stress we apply to it. We do this in the form of lifting weights. As you continue to ask your muscles to move against resistance (lift weights, strength train, resistance training), they have one of two options: move the weight or not move the weight. If your muscles are able to move the resistance easily, then there is no reason to grow or increase in size. But if your muscle either struggles to move against the employed resistance or is unable to at all, it needs to recruit more muscle fibers with the intention to increase the failure threshold. Once you do this, the barriers to meeting your goals are greatly diminished.

> Strength training is the hidden gem that everyone who has successfully lost weight and kept it off is doing.

The body requires energy to do everything. Somewhere there has to be a penance paid for breathing, digestion, sweating, thinking, building muscle, and even eating. More calories are used to make and maintain muscle than fat. Actually the complex systems behind building muscle are some of the largest energy-consuming processes in the entire body. Therefore if you are building muscle, you are in turn requiring the body to use fat as an available energy source. You burn calories during strength training, and your body continues to burn calories after strength training for somewhere between thirty to sixty minutes (although calories burned during exercise represents the most important factor of energy expenditure).[1] In fact, muscle can help to increase your metabolism by up to 15 percent.

The effect of strength training keeps the body running at a high level of energy use during the day. Eating the right foods throughout the day also fuels your metabolism, and any amount that is necessary to repair and increase muscle mass is used, not stored. The benefits are not limited to just daytime activity.

Fat utilization for energy is time dependent, and what better time to pull calories from energy stores than when you are sleeping and not using that stored fat for energy. Once you add in a little aerobic exercise, the muscle you just added helps to improve performance until the heart and lungs can catch up. This pushes you even further toward success as you engage each new exercise bout.

World-class athletes (individuals who possess high percentages of lean muscle mass) can nearly double their daily caloric output with three to four hours of arduous training.[2] They possess the secret ingredient, and with the right level of focus, you can also.

Rita Kubicky and other researchers looked at the long-term effects of nonintensive weight programs on body mass index and metabolic abnormalities in obese children and adolescents. They wanted to know if the data collected for short-term effects of intervention could be reflective of long-term effects by conducting their own four-year study, in which they structured a customized weight management program. They partnered with the Section of Endocrinology and Diabetes at

St. Christopher's Hospital for Children, analyzing changes in BMI (body mass index), glycemic measures (glucose for diabetes), and lipid profiles (cholesterol), along with correlating the changes with the frequency of the followup visits.[3]

A total of sixty-one children and adults were studied, with diet alteration and no more than thirty minutes of continuous activity recommended daily. At the end of four years, the mean average of normal fasting glucose levels dropped by approximately seventeen points, a 7 percent decline was noted in BMI, and 14 percent change in LDL (bad cholesterol). This was done without a heavy focus on weight lifting.

What they were able to find out is that simple, nonintensive weight management programs can be successful with the right amount of monitoring. Imagine how much more effective it would have been if they had injected a little strength training into the equation.

A group of researchers at the University of Massachusetts looked at the metabolic changes associated with the addition of four months of resistive exercise to an existing aerobic exercise program (AEX+RT) as compared to a maintenance aerobic exercise (AEX) in overweight, older men.[4]

Both groups (AEX and AEX+RT) had recently completed a six-month aerobic exercise program using a treadmill walking forty-five minutes a day, two days a week. For the purpose of argument, all clients had some degree of normalized activity level prior to adaptations of the program. The AEX+RT group added six exercises using upper- and lower-body pneumatic-resistance machines such as chest press, shoulder press, bicep curls, leg press, knee extensions, and hamstring curls, while the AEX group continued the same maintenance treadmill AEX program.

Over time, the researchers documented that the insulin responses decreased by 21–29 percent in the AEX+RT group, but did not change at all in the AEX group.[5] They concluded that the addition of resistive exercise training to the existing aerobic exercise program showed promise in improving insulin sensitivity in overweight, older men. Therefore the addition of resistive training could help prevent the development of type 2 diabetes in this specific population.

Major take away point

You need more lean muscle mass to makes things easier, cheating the system. If you lack muscle mass, you make things that much more difficult on yourself. Nobody is saying that you have to put on ten to twenty pounds of muscle to be effective in the weight room, but it will surely lead to increasing your chances of getting the results you are longing for. It is imperative to sway the odds in your favor so that you can meet your goals quicker and beat out the discouragement beast that is currently running you down from behind and ruining all your hard labors and progress toward achieving ultimate health.

CONCLUSION

ARE YOU REALLY ready to take your health seriously? Are you tired of losing the battle? Can you make the significant changes in your life to unlock your true potential and achieve the goals that you should have met ages ago?

Yes, you can! What I have given you in these pages are the tools for success. I've outlined the game plan for exercise, meal modulation, and, most importantly, the spiritual guidance that is imperative to keeping you on course. So what are you waiting for?

God has given me a word of victory to speak over your life right now. You are a spiritual being, living out a human experience. Because of that, you are in an eternal state of transition. You are not stuck in any situation that holds you in bondage. You were fashioned in fire, created in power, and destined in love. You are not stuck in any negative situations. Your perspective is going to make or break you.

I want you to decide today that you are walking in victory. The battle has been won. You are coming out of your circumstances. You are no longer a victim, a loser, a failure, poor, overweight, frustrated, tired, beaten, battered, or sick. You are a rich, energized, passionate, positive thinking victor, and your best days are not behind you but are ahead of you. There are no barriers that you cannot overcome and no mountains too high to climb. The excess weight is coming off of you today. The sickness and disease that had overencumbered you is fleeing from your body as we speak. You blood pressure is normalizing. Your desire for overeating is dissipating.

You crave spiritual food that can build you up and make you mentally ready for the challenge ahead of you. You will not live in doubt anymore, but you will exist in a state of unlimited potential. You are determined to dwell in the place of gain, not loss. Your testimony will help to encourage others and they in turn will do the same for their family and friends.

This is the absolute truth and there is nothing that anyone can say or do about it. You will be better because you have decided to walk in purpose and live on purpose.

Wow! I am so excited for you right now. I know that you have the potential to be so much more than you already are. Everything you need to succeed is already inside of you. Bring a friend along for the journey. Set new standards for the way you want to live. Get the most out of life. Plan your new season and claim the victory today.

Pass up the temptation to put this off for another day while you wait for the perfect circumstances to materialize. Banish those *sinful* ways of the past and look to your new, bright future. Give a little more effort and embrace the power inside you. Turn down the volume and connect to your purpose. Find the time to get it done and realize the strength that will make you a shining testimony of hard work and dedication.

You can make a difference in your life first, and then encourage others to do the same. No excuses, no failures. I can see it already. You are taking the stance and marching toward ultimate health. See you at the finish line!

.

Appendix

ASK THE FAT DOCTOR

Rapid-Fire Bonus Round: A Guide to This Book

I have so many people ask me health-related questions, and it is amazing to know how thirsty people are to learn more about the best ways to take care of themselves. Whether it's at a speaking engagement, health and wellness event, e-mail, blog post, or a question I take on the radio, the one thing I find to be universal is that people are ultimately failing because they are in an information deficit. The best success stories are the ones where I am able to provide a simple answer to a question and unlock that untapped potential in a person. Most times, it's merely as simple as pointing someone in the right direction.

What I have done here in this section of the book is comprise a few questions that I have been asked over the years. I provide the answer to the question, and then refer you (the reader) to the chapter of the book that best reflects the subject matter. Call it a kind of CliffsNotes, Fat Doc style. Enjoy!

Thirty-seven-year-old male asks, "Hey, Fat Doc, how does sleep affect my health?"

A lack of sleep makes you tired. I know that sounds like a weak answer, but it's true. No one can operate functionally and at their maximal capacity on a lack of sleep. The brain needs more sleep than you know. Sleep deprivation negatively affects cognitive function.[1] But it's not limited to just the brain. As a matter of fact, your body needs time to repair itself after a hard bout of exercise in which you have split muscle fibers and fatigued the cardiovascular system. It needs to replenish energy stores and repair these muscles in preparation for the next bout of exercise. Your mental and physical prowess is dependent on the amount of sleep you get on a consistent basis. Most people recommend anywhere between five to ten hours. (Check out chapters 3 and 7.)

Twenty-seven-year-old female asks, "Hey, Fat Doc, how many calories are in a pound?"

I think the question you are asking is how many calories you need to burn in order to lose a pound. But they are kind of one and the same. The general answer is thirty-five hundred kilocalories (kcal). The thing that is important to understand is that different food components contain varying measures of calories. Therefore, one pound of fat contains double the amount of kcal as does the same amount of protein. So, when trying to effectively lose weight, it is best to stay on a low-fat diet, consuming more protein, fiber, and organic acids because they have lower energy densities and increase your chances of losing weight faster. Then, add in exercise to increase the daily caloric expenditures to once again increase your chances of losing weight. Although one size does not fit all, essentially, weight management comes down to one key concept: negative energy balance (fewer calories in and/or more calories out).[2] (Look at chapters 2, 3, 4, and 5.)

Thirty-five-year-old female asks, "Hey, Fat Doc, I heard that working out in the bedroom with your spouse can really help to shed the pounds. Is that true? If so, how often and for how long do you recommend?"

Hey, another thing to remember when trying to lose weight is eat less and move more. Now, movement is movement. For you married folks out there, exercise in the bedroom counts too. And if you're not careful, you might have a good time doing it. Like most exercise programs, it's not about the time your put into it, but the effort. I caution you (as with all exercise prescription) to pace yourself. With that said...I don't want to get in trouble so I will recommend chapters 5, 7, 9 (especially 9), and 10.

Twenty-five-year-old female asks, "Hey, Fat Doc, I have had a lot of health problems since birthing my second child, including heart palpitations, appendicitis, and increased cholesterol (bad stuff—LDL). Are these health problems common? What is a recommended calorie intake for me at my age to successfully lose weight and lower my LDLs?"

STATS! That's covered in *chapter 3*. You can read up on your fitness IQ and the norms to look for concerning cholesterol, blood sugar, and much more. Changes to a woman's body occur after pregnancy due to higher levels of hormones present in the body to help you make it through the child birthing process. Unfortunately, the sky is the limit when it comes to pesky side effects following pregnancy. It is best to report these to your OB-GYN and your primary care physician for their expert advice. But once they clear you for exercise, chapters 2, 5, 7, and 11 should help you along the way.

Fifty-year-old male asks, "Hey, Fat Doc, how many times a week do I really need to do exercises in order to win the battle of the bulge? I do sit-ups like crazy, but the weight just will not move.

Most experts recommend three to four times a week. I recommend having an off day smacked right in the middle for recuperation time both physically and mentally. Also, specificity of exercise is the key, and it sounds like you are focusing on the midsection. That's a good start. But until you trim off the excess weight, you will never see those rock hard abdominal muscles. Concentrate on both diet and exercise to get the maximal results you are looking for. It's important to consider your age as well. Some exercises might be more appropriate than others. You never want to try things that can possibly harm you and set you back even further. Start off easy, navigating the perfect balance between what you do well and maximize that. Then begin to look at those types of exercises that really challenge you. Slowly incorporate those and build as you go. That way you will not become discouraged. Remember, it takes time to see the results, so stay encouraged. (Chapters 7, 12, and 13 will get you on the right track.)

Thirty-seven-year-old female asks, "Hey, Fat Doc, how can I lose inches around my waist and abdominal area? Are fibroids a cause?"

Anything that takes up space in the abdominal cavity can and most likely will strip away the potential of giving you that flat stomach that it sounds like you are searching for. Even the tiniest bit of scarring from surgical procedures or injuries can tighten the fascia and make for protrusions and deformities.

Who wants those? You may want to consult your primary care physician so that he or she can refer you to a gynecologist for options to tackle those fibroids. As for blasting away that fat, chapters 3, 4, and 5 should offer some ideas to ramp up the metabolism and decrease your intake.

Sixty-year-old female asks, "Hey, Fat Doc, I notice that when I don't regularly exercise I tend to get cramps in my muscles. What can I do to prevent the cramping if I don't have time to get the exercise in?"

Your diet will be a key ingredient to solving the muscle cramps. Staying hydrated (especially in the winter months) is a huge issue as we age. Our bodies become more and more inflexible, as we lose both water and muscle mass (contractile tissue) over time. It is important to stretch more frequently, longer than normal (both before and after exercise), and continue to pump our bodies with vitamins and nutrients that aid in the maintenance process. Look to chapters 5 and 7 for food choices and exercise prescriptions.

Be safe, everyone!

NOTES

Introduction
Breaking Cycles of Defeat

1. Katherine M. Flegal et al., "Prevalence and Trends in Obesity Among US Adults, 1999–2008," *Journal of the American Medical Association* 303, no. 3 (January 20, 2010): 235–241.

2. Ibid.

3. Ibid.

4. Kylie Wilson and Darren Brookfield, "Effect of Goal Setting on Motivation and Adherence in a Six-Week Exercise Program," *International Journal of Sport and Exercise Physiology*, 6, no. 1 (March 2009): 89–100, as cited in Len Kravitz, "Exercise Motivation: What Starts and Keeps People Exercising?," http://www .unm.edu/~lkravitz/Article%20folder/ExerciseMot.pdf (accessed August 22, 2014).

5. Cora Lynne Craig, Christine Cameron, Storm J. Russell, and Angèle Beaulieu, "Increasing Physical Activity: Supporting Children's Participation," Canadian Fitness and Lifestyle Research Institute, http://www.cflri.ca/media/node/422/ files/2000pam.pdf (accessed August 26, 2014).

Chapter 1
Claim Success for a New Season

1. Arlene K. Unger, "Can Positive Thinking Help With Weight Loss?," *Real Psych Solutions*, http://www.realpsychsolutions.com/ uploads/Can-Positive-Thinking-Help-with-Weight-Loss-rps.pdf (accessed November 3, 2014).

2. Brenda W. J. H. Penninx et al., "Changes in Depression and Physical Decline in Older Adults: A Longitudinal Perspective," *Journal of Affective Disorders* 61 (2000): 1–12.

Chapter 2
Recognize and Move Past Your Obstacles

1. Douglas Carroll et al., "Cardiovascular Reactions to Psychological Stress: The Influence of Demographic Variables," *Journal of Epidemiological Community Health* 54 (2000): 876–877.

2. A. Appels and P. Mulder, "Fatigue and Heart Disease: The Association Between 'Vital Exhaustion' and Past, Present and Future Coronary Heart Disease," *Journal of Psychosomatic Research* 33, no. 6 (1989): 727–738.

3. N. Chumaeva et al., "Interactive Effect of Long-Term Mental Stress and Cardiac Stress Reactivity on Carotid Intima-Media Thickness: The Cardiovascular Risk in Young Finns Study," *Stress* 12, no. 4 (July 2009): 283–293.

Chapter 3
All You Need to Succeed Is You

1. This material on Wilma Rudolph has been adapted from her autobiography: *Wilma Rudolph, The Story of Wilma Rudolph* (New York: New American Library, 1977).

2. Preamble to the Constitution of the World Health Organization as adopted by the International Health Conference, New York, 19-22 June, 1946; signed on July 22, 1946 by the representatives of sixty-one states (Official Records of the World Health Organization, no. 2, 100) and entered into force on April 7, 1948.

3. Merriam-Webster.com, s.v. "wellness," http://www.merriam-webster.com/dictionary/wellness (accessed November 3, 2014).

4. To review additional information related to the President's Council on Physical Fitness and Sports, see "Definitions: Health, Fitness, and Physical Activity," https://www.presidentschallenge.org/informed/digest/docs/200003digest.pdf (accessed November 3, 2014).

5. C. Cooper, G. Campion, and L. J. Melton III, "Hip Fractures in the Elderly: A World-Wide Projection," *Osteoporosis International* 2, no. 6 (November 1992): 285–289.

6. D. L. Ballor and R. E. Keesey, "A Meta-Analysis of the Factors Affecting Exercise-Induced Changes in Body Mass, Fat Mass, and Fat-Free Mass in Males and Females," *International Journal of Obesity* 15, no. 11 (1991): 717–726.

7. P. Arner, E. Kriegholm, P. Engfeldt, and J. Bolinder, "Adrenergic Regulation of Lipolysis in Situ at Rest and During Exercise," Journal of Clinical Investigation 85, no. 3 (March 1990): 893–898; R. S. Schwartz et al., "The Effect of Intensive Endurance Exercise Training on Body Fat Distribution in Young and Older Men," *Metabolism* 40, no. 5 (May 1991): 545–551; M. A. Staten, "The Effect of Exercise on Food Intake in Men and Women," *American Journal of Clinical Nutrition* 53, no. 1 (January 1991): 27–31; H. Wahrenberg, J. Bolinder, P. Arner, "Adrenergic Regulation of Lipolysis in Human Fat Cells During Exercise," *European Journal of Clinical Investigation* 21, no. 5 (October 1991): 534–541.

8. Merriam-Webster.com, s.v. "metabolism," http://www.merriam-webster.com/dictionary/metabolism (accessed September 5, 2014).

9. Ibid.

Chapter 4
Sins of the Father

1. Goodreads.com, "Ella Fitzgerald Quotes," http://www.goodreads.com/quotes/66511-it-isn-t-where-you-came-from-it-s-where-you-re-going (accessed November 4, 2014).

2. EurekAlert, "Essential Nutrient Found in Eggs Reduces Risk of Breast Cancer By 24 Percent," *Edelman Public Relations*, April 3, 2008, http://www.eurekalert.org/pub_releases/2008-04/epr-enf040208.php (accessed November 3, 2014).

3. Xavier Pi-Sunyer, "The Medical Risks of Obesity," *Postgraduate Medicine* 121, no. 6 (November 2009): 21–33.

4. Katherine M. Flegal, Margaret D. Carroll, Cynthia L. Ogden, and Lester R. Curtin, "Prevalence and Trends in Obesity Among US Adults, 1999–2008," *Journal of the American Medical Association* 303, no. 3 (2010): 235–241.

5. Cynthia L. Ogden, Molly M. Lamb, Margaret D. Carroll, and Katherine M. Flegal, "Obesity and Socioeconomic Status in Adults: United States, 2005–2008," *National Center for Health Statistics*, no. 50 (December 2010).

Chapter 5
Turn Down the Volume and Liste

1. Roderick J. Flower, "Drugs Which Inhibit Prostaglandin Biosynthesis," *Pharmacological Reviews* 26, no. 1 (March 1974): 33–67.

2. Alan Aragon, Alan's Vault, http://alanaragon.com/ (accessed September 5, 2014).

3. Alan Aragon's Calorie Calculator equation is cited in Ben Court, "Is Exercise Fattening?" *Men's Health* (October 2012): 102–107. The author cited from the printed article, and it can also be accessed at http://business.highbeam.com/435920/article -1G1-313753542/exercise-fattening (accessed September 5, 2014).

Chapter 6
It You're Not Giving, Then You're Not Getting

1. Edward Chaney, "Egypt in England and America: The Cultural Memorials of Religion, Royalty and Revolution," in *Sites of Exchange: European Crossroads and Faultlines*, Maurizio Ascari and Adriana Corrado, eds. (Amsterdam and New York: Rodopi BV, 2006), 39–74.

2. "Report on Medical Care," *British National Archives* (WO 33/1 ff.119, 124, 146–7). Dated February 23, 1855.

3. Cited in Edward Tyas Cook, *The Life of Florence Nightingale*, vol. 1 (London: Macmillan and Co., Limited, 1913), 237.

Chapter 7
Embrace Your Power

1. Lydia Ievleva and Terry Orlick, "Mental Links to Enhanced Healing: An Exploratory Study," *The Sports Psychologist* 5 (1991): 25–40.
2. Michael N. Mavros et al., "Do Psychological Variables Affect Early Surgical Recovery?," *PLoS One* 6, no. 5 (2011):e20306.

Chapter 8
Connect With Your Purpose

1. This takeaway is presented courtesy of a sermon by Dr. Mark Rutland.
2. Richard B. Kreider et al., "A Structured Diet and Exercise Program Promotes Favorable Changes in Weight Loss, Body Composition, and Weight Maintenance," *Journal of the American Dietetic Association* 111, no. 6 (June 2011): 828–843.
3. Ibid.

Chapter 9
Buddy Up

1. Thomas G. Plante et al. "Exercising With an iPod, Friend, or Neither: Which Is Better for Psychological Benefits?" *American Journal of Health Behavior* 35, no. 2 (March–April 2011): 199–208.
2. Thomas G. Plante et al., "Effects of Perceived Fitness Level of Exercise Partner on Intensity of Exertion," *Journal of Social Sciences* 6, no. 1 (2010): 50–54.

Chapter 10
Get Moving

1. Brian E. Udermann et al., "Spirituality in the Curricula of Accredited Athletic Training Education Programs," *Athletic Training Education Journal* 1 (January–March 2008): 21–27.

2. D. B. Larson et al., "The Impact of Religion on Men's Blood Pressure," *Journal of Religion and Health* 28, no. 4 (December 1989): 265–278.

3. G. W. Comstock and K. B. Partridge, "Church Attendance and Health," *Journal of Chronic Diseases* 25, no. 12 (December 1972): 665–672.

4. D. M. Zuckerman, S. V. Kasl, and A. M. Ostfield, "Psychosocial Predictors of Mortality Among the Elderly Poor: The Role of Religion, Well-Being, and Social Contacts," *American Journal of Epidemiology* 119, no. 3 (March 1984): 410–423.

5. J. A. Roberts, D. Brown, T. Elkins, and D. B. Larson, "Factors Influencing Views of Patients With Gynecologic Cancer About End-of-Life Decisions," *American Journal of Obstetrics and Gynecology* 176 (January 1997): 166–172.

6. R. Casar Harris et al., "The Role of Religion in Heart -Transplant Recipients' Long-Term Health and Well-Being," *Journal of Religion and Health* 34, no. 1 (March 1995): 17–32.

7. R. C. Byrd, "Positive Therapeutic Effects of Intercessory Prayer in a Coronary Care Unit Population," *Southern Medical Journal* 81, no. 7 (July 1988): 826–829.

8. H. G. Koenig, "Religion, Spirituality, and Medicine: Application to Clinical Practice," *Journal of the American Medical Association* 284, no. 13 (October 4, 2000): 1708.

9. L. N. Robins et al., "Lifetime Prevalence of Specific Psychiatric Disorders in Three Sites," *Archives of General Psychiatry* 41, no. 10 (October 1984): 949–958.

10. A. W. Braam et al., "Religiosity as a Protective or Prognostic Factor of Depression in Later Life; Results From a Community Survey in the Netherlands," *Acta Psychiatrica Scandinavica* 96, no. 3 (September 1997): 199–205.

11. J. M. Kaczorowski, "Spiritual Well-Being and Anxiety in Adults Diagnosed With Cancer," *Hospice Journal* 5, no. 3–4 (1989): 105–116.

12. Ibid.

13. R. L. Gorsuch, M.C. Butler, "Initial Drug Abuse: A Review of Predisposing Social Psychological Factors," *Psychological Bulletin* 83, no. 1 (1976): 120–137; J. D. Hovey, "Religion and Suicidal

Ideation in a Sample of Latin American Immigrants," *Psychological Reports* 85, no. 1 (August 1999): 171–177; S. Stack and D. Lester, "The Effect of Religion on Suicide Ideation," *Social Psychiatry and Psychiatric Epidemiology* 26, no. 4 (August 1991): 168–170.

14. M. Siegrist, "Church Attendance, Denomination, and Suicide Ideology," *Journal of Social Psychology* 136, no. 5 (October 1996): 559–566.

15. Ibid.; H. G. Koenig, M. E. McCullough, and D. B. Larson, *Handbook of Religion and Health* (New York: Oxford University Press, 2001); D. B. Larson, J. P. Swyers, and M. E. McCullough, Scientific Research on Spirituality and Health: a Report Based on the Scientific Progress in Spirituality Conferences (Rockville, MD: National Institute for Healthcare Research, 1998).

16. Kevin S. Seybold and Peter C. Hill, "The Role of Religion and Spirituality in Mental and Physical Health," *Current Directions in Psychological Science* 10 (2001): 21–24.

17. Luciano Bernardi et al., "Effect of Rosary Prayer and Yoga Mantras on Autonomic Cardiovascular Rhythms: Comparative Study," *British Medical Journal* 323 (2001): 1446–1449.

18. Ibid.

19. M. A. Testa, D. C. Simonson, "Assessment of Quality-Of-Life Outcomes," *New England Journal of Medicine* 334, no. 13 (March 28, 1996): 835–840; Dale A. Matthews, David B. Larson, and Constance P. Barry, The Faith Factor: An Annotated Bibliography of Clinical Research on Spiritual Subjects (Volume 1) (Rockville, MD: National Institute for Healthcare Research, 1993); J. J. Mytko, S. J. Knight, "Body, Mind and Spirit: Towards the Integration of Religiosity and Spirituality in Cancer Quality of Life Research," *Psychooncology* 8, no. 5 (September–October 1999): 439–450; B. B. Riley et al., "Types of Spiritual Well-Being Among Persons with Chronic Illness: Their Relation to Various Forms of Quality of Life," *Archives of Physical Medicine and Rehabilitation* 79, no. 3 (March 1998): 258–264; Luciano Bernardi et al., "Effect of Rosary Prayer and Yoga Mantras on Autonomic Cardiovascular Rhythms: Comparative Study."

20. S. P. Cotton, E. G. Levine, C. M. Fitzpatrick et al., "Exploring the Relationships Among Spiritual Well-Being, Quality of Life, and Psychological Adjustment in Women with Breast Cancer," *Psychooncology* 8, no. 5 (September–October 1999): 429–438; M. J. Brady et al., "A Case for Including Spirituality in Quality of Life Measurement in Oncology," *Psychooncology* 8, no. 5 (September–October 1999): 417–428.

21. Luciano Bernardi et al., "Effect of Rosary Prayer and Yoga Mantras on Autonomic Cardiovascular Rhythms: Comparative Study."

Chapter 11
There Are No Perfect Circumstances

1. Douglas Brooks, *Effective Strength Training: Analysis and Technique for Upper-Body, Lower-Body, and Trunk Exercises* (n.p.: Human Kinetics, 2001), 51–52.

2. Ibid.

3. Ibid.

4. Jerrold Petrofsky et al., "Muscle Use During Isometric Co-contraction of Agonist-Antagonist Muscle Pairs in the Upper and Lower Body Compared to Abdominal Crunches and a Commercial Multi Gym Exerciser," *Journal of Applied Research* 6, no. 4 (2006): 300–328.

5. A. V. Hill, "The Pressure Developed in Muscle During Contraction," *Journal of Physiology* 107 (1948): 518–526; R. H. Edwards, D. K. Hill and M. McDonnell, "Myothermal and Intramuscular Pressure Measurements During Isometric Contractions of the Human Quadriceps Muscle," *Journal of Physiology* 224, no. 2 (July 1972): 58P–59P.

6. H. Barcroft and J. E. Millen, "Blood Flow Through Muscle During Sustained Contraction," *Journal of Physiology* 97, no. 1 (November 14, 1939): 17–31.

7. J. P. Folland et al., "Strength Training: Isometric Training at a Range of Joint Angles Versus Dynamic Training," *Journal of Sports Sciences* 23, no. 8 (August 2005): 817–824; S. J. Fleck and

R. C. Schutt Jr, "Types of Strength Training," *Orthopedic Clinics of North America* 14, no. 2 (April 1983): 449–458.

8. N. Rahnama, A. Lees, and T. Reilly, "Electromyography of Selected Lower-Limb Muscles Fatigued by Exercise at the Intensity of Soccer Match-Play," *Journal of Electromyography and Kinesiology* 16, no. 3 (June 2006): 257–263.

9. Ibid.

10. Manuel Monfort-Pañego et al., "Abdominal Exercises Review," *Journal of Manipulative and Physiological Therapeutics* (March/April 2009): 232–244.

Chapter 12
Broken Clock

1. Rena R. Wing and James O. Hill, "Successful Weight Loss Maintenance," *Annual Review of Nutrition* 21 (2001): 323–341.

2. Ibid.

3. J. Kassirer and M. Angell, "Losing Weight: An Ill-Fated New Year's Resolution," *New England Journal of Medicine* 338, no. 1 (January 1998): 52–54.

4. A. J. Stunkard and M. McLaren-Hume, "The Results of Treatment for Obesity," *Archives of Internal Medicine* 103 (1959): 79–85.

5. K. D. Brownell, "Whether Obesity Should Be Treated," *Health Psychology* 12, no. 5 (September 1993): 339–341; K. D. Brownell and J. Rodin, "Medical, Metabolic, and Psychological Effects of Weight Cycling," *Archives of Internal Medicine* 154, no. 12 (June 1994): 1325–1330.

6. M. L. Klem et al., "A Descriptive Study of Individuals Successful at Long-Term Maintenance of Substantial Weight Loss," *American Journal of Clinical Nutrition* 66, no. 2 (August 1997): 239–246.

7. Raymond C. Baker and Daniel S. Kirschenbaum, "Self-Monitoring May Be Necessary for Successful Weight Control," *Behavior Therapy* 24, no. 3 (1993): 377–394.

Chapter 13
Realize Your Strength

1. William D. McArdle, Frank I. Katch and Victor L. Katch, *Sports and Exercise Nutrition* (Philadelphia, PA: Lippincott Williams and Wilkins, 1999), 444–446.

2. Ibid.

3. Rita Ann Kubicky et al., "Long-Term Effects of a Non-Intensive Weight Program on Body Mass in Metabolic Abnormalities of Obese Children and Adolescents," *International Journal of Pediatric Endocrinology* 2012 (2012): 16.

4. C. M. Ferrara et al., "Metabolic Effects of the Addition of Resistive to Aerobic Exercise in Older Men," *International Journal of Sport Nutrition and Exercise Metabolism* 14, no. 1 (February 2004): 73–80.

5. Ibid.

Appendix
Ask the Fat Doctor

1. M. Skein et al., "The Effect of Overnight Sleep Deprivation Following Competitive Rugby League Matches on Postmatch Physiological and Perceptual Recovery," *International Journal of Sports Physiology and Performance* 8, no. 5 (September 2013): 556–564.

2. L. E. Shay et al., "Adult Weight Management: Translating Research and Guidelines Into Practice," *Journal of the American Academy of Nurse Practitioners* 21, no. 4 (2009): 197–206.

About the Author

Dr. Braxton A. Cosby, CEO of Cosby Media Productions, is a dreamer who plays around with ideas in his mind that he desires to bring to life in print and share with the entire world. Braxton is an eternal student who ventures to learn more and more each day and embraces the idea of facing challenges head on, accomplishing what people determine as impossible. Braxton has used his experience as a physical therapist, certified nutritionist and personal trainer, to encourage people to get moving and experience life to the fullest by achieving their personal fitness goals. Braxton is also an award-winning author of young adult and sci-fi novels. Braxton is married, has three lovely girls, and currently resides in Georgia.

Follow Braxton:
www.braxtoncosby.com

Twitter:
@BraxtonACosby

Facebook:
www.facebook.com/DrBraxtonCosby

Author Organization

Braxton is a member of Tabernacle International Church in Lawrenceville, Georgia, under the teachings of Apostle Fritz Musser and Lady Lisa Musser.

Cosby Media Productions (CMP): a full-service media group that focuses on producing content across various platforms such as print, music, television and film. CMP desires to "Educate the Mind and Inspire the Soul" through providing uplifting, family-friendly content to the masses.

Catch up with CMP @ www.cosbymediaproductions.com

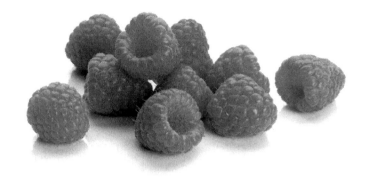
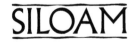

Made in the USA
San Bernardino, CA
05 January 2016